LIVING MEDICINE
Planning a career: choosing a specialty

T0292119

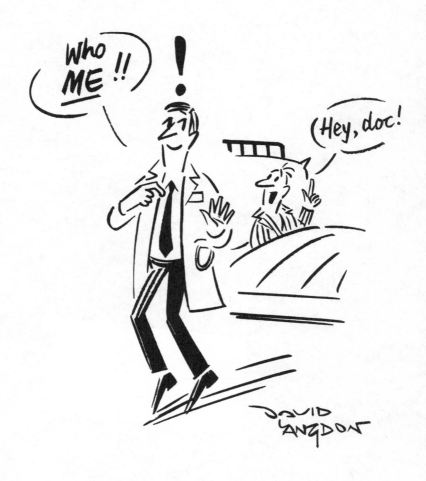

... sooner than they think ...

LIVING MEDICINE
Planning a career: choosing a specialty

PETER RICHARDS MA MD PHD FRCP

Professor of Medicine and Dean
St Mary's Hospital Medical School

and

ProRector (Medicine)
Imperial College of Science, Technology and Medicine
University of London

with line drawings by

DAVID LANGDON OBE FRSA

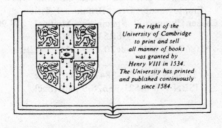

*The right of the
University of Cambridge
to print and sell
all manner of books
was granted by
Henry VIII in 1534.
The University has printed
and published continuously
since 1584.*

CAMBRIDGE UNIVERSITY PRESS
Cambridge
New York   Port Chester
Melbourne   Sydney

CAMBRIDGE UNIVERSITY PRESS
Cambridge, New York, Melbourne, Madrid, Cape Town, Singapore, São Paulo, Delhi

Cambridge University Press
The Edinburgh Building, Cambridge CB2 8RU, UK

Published in the United States of America by Cambridge University Press, New York

www.cambridge.org
Information on this title: www.cambridge.org/9780521386289

First published 1990
Re-issued in this digitally printed version 2009

A catalogue record for this publication is available from the British Library

Library of Congress Cataloguing in Publication data
Richards, Peter, M.D.
Living medicine.   Planning a career: choosing a specialty /
Peter Richards: with line drawings by David Langdon.
p.   cm.
Includes bibliographical references.
ISBN 0–521–38478–8. – ISBN 0–521–38628–4 (pbk.)
1. Medicine – Specialties and specialists – Great Britain.
2. Medicine – Vocational guidance – Great Britain.   3. Physicians –
Employment – Great Britain.   I. Title.
[DNLM: 1. Career Choice.   2. Specialties, Medical.   W 90 R513L]
R7Z9.5.S6R53   1990
610.69´52´0941—dc20   89–25175   CIP

ISBN 978-0-521-38478-0 hardback
ISBN 978-0-521-38628-9 paperback

The British Government have announced that they intend to establish a comprehensive Health Service for everyone in the country. They want to ensure that in future every man, woman and child can rely on getting all the advice, treatment and care which they may need in matters of personal health; that what they will get will be the best medicine and other facilities available; that their getting them shall not depend on whether they can pay for them, or on any factor irrelevant to the real need – the real need to bring the country's full resources to bear upon reducing ill-health and promoting good health for all its citizens.

Sir John Hawton, 1944

Contents

vii

Preface

Medicine soon becomes a way of life: satisfying and rewarding, tiring and demanding, especially for those with domestic responsibilities. The attractions are transparent but the personal cost is less obvious. Most doctors would not change their job for another, but a few would (and do) and many have had moments of disillusionment, partly because they were not adequately prepared for the difficulties.

Learning Medicine[1] was written for those thinking of applying to medical school. *Living Medicine*, its sequel, attempts to prepare senior students and house officers for their responsibilities and opportunities as doctors: for the reality that qualification is only the beginning of an exciting but hard road. It may, however, also be a useful supplement to *Learning Medicine* at the outset: not fully intelligible to those unfamiliar with clinical medicine but clear enough in its message that a career in medicine not only enriches but also dominates life.

My warmest thanks are due to many colleagues who have increased my knowledge of their own specialties and of the preparation for them. Any inspired glimpses of the diversity of medicine are theirs; any undeserved dullness or errors are mine. If my tone seems cautious that caution does not indicate lack of enthusiasm for a career second to none, only the belief that the best medicine for difficulties in life and work is to be ready for them.

Peter Richards
St Mary's Hospital Medical School
Imperial College

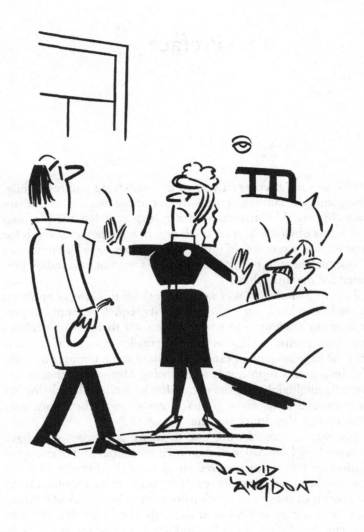

. . . a danger to patients . . .

I

What becomes of medical students?

Almost all medical students become doctors, and sooner than they think. About 6% of those who start fail to qualify, most because of academic failure in the preclinical years where, normally, only two attempts at the examinations are permitted at each stage. A few fall by the wayside later because they lose heart, interest or health. A very small number fail to graduate on the three or four attempts at Finals which their universities permit them, during which time they are also able to sit for nonuniversity diplomas which qualify them to practise.

The perpetual student has become a memory of the past. With a sufficient number of attempts, particularly if taken single subject by single subject, most medical students would pass; that is not the object of the exercise. Qualification (by degree or diploma) to practise is a demonstration within a reasonable time (generally within two years of completion of the clinical course) of a standard of competence, knowledge and attitude such that the individual seems safe, sensible, stable and able to continue to learn from experience.

Both reason and experience indicate that under all normal conditions anyone who has completed a university course of between five and six years and has not within two years of finishing the course passed a qualifying examination, has failed to integrate the knowledge gained so as to apply it to practical problems of patients. Such a person is not only likely to have difficulty and distress in long years of postgraduate training but may possibly be a danger to patients. The welfare of patients is as proper a concern of medical schools as the aspirations of their students; when, as happens from time to time, the one must be balanced against the other, the interests of the patient must surely win. Once qualified to practise there is no effective recognition of incompetence in the medical profession until either a patient is harmed or behaviour is outrageously unprofessional; that is too late.

What doctors eventually become and why is relatively easy to discover. Whether a medical student turns into a good doctor is much more difficult to determine, not least because there are no agreed objective measures. Professional success can be assessed academically, economically and, perhaps, politically but expertise and patient satisfaction are problematic.

Career preferences

The great majority of home graduates in medicine now make their career in the UK. The days of substantial medical emigration of UK graduates to North America, Australia and New Zealand are over. Almost all doctors in the UK work for the National Health Service (NHS) directly or in an honorary capacity in a university post; only about 2% of doctors registered in and resident in the UK work entirely outside the NHS.

Most doctors work in general practice or in hospital specialties; approximately twice as many permanent career posts are in general practice as in hospital (Table 1.1). About 8% of doctors find career posts within community medicine (public health) and related specialties.

Over 90% of medical graduates continue in medicine, three-quarters of them working fulltime for most of their working

Table 1.1. Principals in general practice and consultants in hospital practice in England and Wales, 1987[2]

Specialty	Number in permanent, senior career posts
General practice	26 678
Hospital practice	14 800

lives. A survey of graduates of 1966, 1976 and 1981 showed that 75% were working fulltime and 19% part-time in 1986. Half of the latter were in general practice, one-quarter in hospital specialities and more than half the remainder in community medicine; at the time of survey all the men and 60% of the women were working fulltime[3].

Finding a niche takes time, sometimes a long time. Career preferences at the end of the pre-registration year for paediatrics, general medicine, general surgery, obstetrics and gynaecology and anaesthetics exceed opportunity. Career posts in pathology and radiology correspond to the proportion of doctors seeking them. Fewer doctors at that moment in their career are intending to specialise in psychiatry, general practice and, especially, in community medicine than the number needed to fill the career-training posts available (Table 1.2)

Over the next few years between one-quarter and one-third of graduates change their choices, some more than once. Initial career intentions are shaped partly by experience as a student and house officer and partly on a rather hazy perception of prospects in different specialties. Domestic responsibilities receive little weight at this stage, because most doctors are still unmarried and do not come to terms with the fact that most will marry over the next few years. Final career decisions are based on an increasingly realistic assessment of career opportunity and other responsibilities: about 40% change because of family commitments, including 60% of women with children. Twice as many women as men referred to marriage as a career constraint in Allen's survey, but it was mentioned by 25% of men.[3]

It is possible to calculate the number of graduates who can enter any particular specialty and secure a permanent post within a reasonable time. It is much more difficult to predict the precise number of posts which will become vacant in a defined period because of a fluctuating pattern of retirement. Further, posts may be abolished on retirement to save money. On the other hand, more consultant posts have been promised. Even if a sufficient expansion materialises the specialty mix of new posts in any particular period is currently unpredictable. Whatever the ambition it is necessary to remain domestically mobile until a permanent post is secured.

Table 1.2. Career first preference towards the end of the
preregistration year in relation to available career posts in
1980[4]

Career	% of graduates	% of permanent career posts	Ratio of intention to opportunity
Clinical practice outside hospital			
General practice	37	58	0.6
Clinical practice in hospital			
General medicine and medical specialties	18	7	2.6
General surgery and surgical specialties	16	8	2.0
Anaesthesia	6	4	1.5
Paediatrics	5	1	5.0
Obstetrics and gynaecology	4	2	2.0
Psychiatry	4	5	0.8
Radiotherapy/oncology	1	<1	≈1.0
Clinical support services in hospital			
Pathology	4	4	1.0
Radiology	2	2	1.0
Community medicine	1	8	0.1
Other careers or undecided	2	–	–

Subsequent surveys, including the University Hospitals Association survey in 1987[5] of graduates of 1981, 1983 and 1985 show a similar pattern of choice but with an increased interest in general practice and reduction in both general medicine and surgery and their subspecialties.

Achieving a balance

Central to current planning is the manifesto *Hospital Medical Staffing: Achieving a Balance – Plan for Action* published in 1987 on behalf of the UK Health Departments, the Joint Consultants Committee and Chairmen of Regional Health Authorities.[6] There is wide agreement with its aim to relate career training posts to the number of permanent senior posts but concern, particularly amongst senior doctors about some of its effects. Junior staff will be substantially reduced, training programmes will probably become increasingly rigid and opportunities for training in research will be restricted. The nature of consultant work will inevitably change; clearly it is in the public interest that a larger proportion of hospital services should be provided by fully trained and experienced senior doctors but it cannot happen without abandoning the traditional role of all senior doctors as consultants (see Chapter 3). While being cautious about the extent to which future consultant posts may resemble current senior registrar posts, trainees generally accept an inevitable change in the responsibilities of senior doctors as an acceptable price to pay for a more predictable training pathway and earlier appointment to a permanent post. *Achieving a Balance* is the first concerted attempt since the introduction of the NHS to tackle (over a period of 10 years) the serious imbalance between training posts, of which there are too many, and career posts, of which there are too few. While the principles underlying the *Plan for Action* are exemplary, putting them into practice will be more difficult. The aims are shown in Table 1.3.

Table 1.3. Aims of *Achieving a Balance*

---

1. An increase in the number of consultants, to provide both the leadership and the career opportunities an expanding service requires.

2. Sensible planning of the numbers of doctors in training grades, taking account of career prospects.

3. Maintenance of the necessary levels of support for consultants, especially those in the acute specialties.

The planning process will require a 40% reduction in the number of registrar posts to correct the substantial excess of registrar posts (held for two or three years) over senior registrar posts (held for about four years), which over 10 years will revolutionise the way in which the hospital service is provided. Hitherto a large influx of overseas doctors (now rapidly declining), who spent several years in registrar posts while working for a higher qualification before returning home has concealed the extent of the problems. Even so, some doctors planning a career in the UK have spent many years in the registrar grade without any

realistic prospect of promotion. More would have run aground
had training requirements in different specialties in the past not
been sufficiently flexible to permit sideways moves between hospital specialties and between hospital and general practice.

This flexibility is disappearing as it becomes increasingly
necessary to commit oneself to a particular specialty training at an
early stage. Career pathways will be firmly determined in future
from the beginning of the registrar grade. Indeed the eventual
amalgamation of the registrar and senior registrar grades into one
training grade is envisaged. This would steer a recently qualified
doctor, if not from cradle to grave, at least from completion of
senior house officer (SHO) posts to consultancy or a principalship
in general practice on one tramline. The advantages of the predict-
ability of such a scheme have to be set against the difficulty of
stepping aside to gain diverse experience at home or abroad, or
for a period of research training and the difficulty of changing
one's mind.

Arrangements for registrar posts are these: the total number of
registrar posts will first be determined by career opportunity. An
academic and research quota will be top-sliced and split between
clinical academic and research posts by an Academic and
Research Sub-Group of a central Joint Planning Advisory
Committee (JPAC). The research quota is not specialty-specific
but the academic posts are, and will be divided between regions
by the Sub-Group. The academic quota for each region will
then be subdivided locally between the medical schools. The
remaining 'career' registrar posts will be divided between regions
by JPAC.

Medical Research Council funded posts are in a category of
their own. A separate quota will also be given to the Association
of Medical Research Charities (AMRC), which will be divided
between their member charities. A small number of uncommitted
research posts funded by bodies such as pharmaceutical
companies will also be allocated to regions.

'Visiting' registrars, 'stuck doctors' and the 'nontraining' grade

Doctors eligible to pursue a career in the UK will compete for
'career' registrar posts after one, two or perhaps several years as

an SHO. Overseas doctors not entitled to stay for more than four years of postgraduate training will be eligible for 'visiting' registrar posts which are required to be equally valuable training posts. It is recognised that some doctors will for one reason or another, progress so far and no further ('stuck doctors'), and steps are to be taken to identify and counsel them.

A new 'non-training' grade is to be introduced in the hospital service, partly for those who in future do not progress in a reasonable time from SHO to registrar or who do not seek consultant responsibility.

While the plan provides for a safety net of junior staff at each acute hospital it seems almost inevitable that it will not be possible to provide acute services in as many hospitals as at present. Without an increased number of senior staff to take over part of their duties it would seem that the reduced junior staff would be so fully stretched with essential service tasks that little time would remain for teaching students, for continuing their own postgraduate education and for research. The extent to which 'visiting' registrars may fill the gap remains to be seen.

Senior registrar posts

Steps are successfully in hand to tailor the number of senior registrar posts to consultant retirements and to distribute these posts throughout the UK to regions on the advice of the central Joint Planning Advisory Committee, 'Joint' between the Department of Health, the British Medical Association (BMA), the Royal Colleges, Universities, Research Councils and other interests. Regional committees have distributed the posts within regions. The intention of providing the best possible training posts while ensuring that their teaching and service functions are honoured seems generally to have been achieved. Senior registrars can in future expect to obtain a consultant post within about four years, although they will need to regard the whole country as their oyster, to an even greater extent than in the past.

An expansion of the consultant grade by 2% per annum is crucial to the success of the plan, partly to re-provide services formerly undertaken by junior staff and partly to secure earlier promotion to a permanent post.

Measures of success

Whatever the qualities needed for the many different tasks in medicine the ability to communicate well both with colleagues and patients is fundamental. If interviews in the selection for medical school tell nothing else they should succeed in identifying the good communicators. As far as potential is concerned, an Australian physiologist recently likened medical students to race horses; no amount of physiological, anatomical, psychological, educational, cultural or even genetic scrutiny proves potential. At the end of the day the only measure of a race horse which counts is the ability to win races. Which perhaps means that professional success, is the nearest, if imperfect, proxy to the good doctor, accepting that a few good doctors may not be professionally successful and that some charlatans will win more fame and fortune than their knowledge and skill justifies. The fact that different qualities are required to achieve success in different specialties is one of the great attractions of medicine as a career.

Sir James Paget, one of the Victorian giants of surgery, was perhaps the first person to try to audit the outcome of medical education. He followed the careers of 1000 students between 10 and 15 years after their entry to St Bartholomew's Hospital in the first half of the nineteenth century. His categories of outcome are summarised in Table 1.4.

Table 1.4. Success achieved by 1000 students of
St Bartholomew's Hospital between 1839 and 1869 within
10–15 years of entry[7]

Degree of success	Number
Distinguished	23
Considerable	66
Fair	507
Limited	124
Failed entirely	56
Left the profession	96
Died within 12 years of commencing practice	87
Died as students	41

By 'distinguished' he meant those now maintaining leading practices in countries or large towns, holding important public offices, or working as the medical officers of large hospitals. To these he added 'teachers in great schools', for example the Professors of Anatomy in Oxford, Cambridge and Edinburgh, 'all of whom it was my singular good fortune to have for pupils'. 'Considerable success' applied to those who gained and 'still hold' high positions in the public services, leading practices in good districts or who had already retired on money earned in practice! Included also were those who had gained 'more than ordinary esteem and influence in society'. 'Fair success' described those with 'a fair practice – enough to live with – maintaining a good professional and personal reputation, or in holding ordinary appointments in the public services, or in the colonies, and gaining promotion in due course'. 'Very limited success' was a matter of just hanging on, with little prospect of promotion, 'just living, and that not well, by their work' – in a nutshell, 'doing much less than, with their education and other opportunities of success, they should have achieved'. Little good can be said of those who had 'failed entirely', a disparate bunch 'agreeing only in their total want of success'. They included 15 who never passed their examinations and of those who had passed, 5 had been guilty of scandalous misconduct, 10 had given up because of ill-health or misfortune, 'sheer ill-luck, it seemed', and an equal number had come to grief because of 'the same habits of intemperance or dissipation as had made us even while they were students, anticipate their failure'.

About 10% of the whole group had left the profession altogether over the period, some who had 'left or were expelled in disgrace', a few 'wisely removed by their friends', two retired on private means 'too rich to need to work', a few who had run into trouble of one sort or another as doctors (one 'rather sinned against than sinning') and another 'who had been a good student, speculated in mines, lost money, forged and is in prison'. Many had gone into other professions including the army, the church, the Law, business, farming, the stage (including one 'well esteemed in gentile comedy') and even three who became homeopathic practitioners 'but took to that class no repute for either wisdom or working power'.

The range of success is as wide today as it was then; failure is less colourful and fewer leave for other walks of life. Most different of all is the mortality (128 had died), accounting for 13% of Paget's series, 4% even before qualification. He noted, however, that life tables predicted that out of 1000 males (and all his students were males) attaining the age of 19 years, 131 would die within 15 years. Paget concluded that 'the number agrees so nearly with the general average mortality that it gives no reason for considering the medical profession either less or more healthy than other pursuits, at least in its earlier stages'. Taking into account the upper class origins of the students and their otherwise less than average mortality this surely implies that students and doctors risked their health in serving their patients. To learn through serving, even at personal risk, is one thing which still happens to medical students.

2
Clinical freedom and professional responsibility

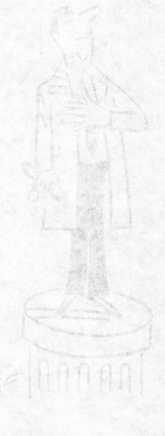

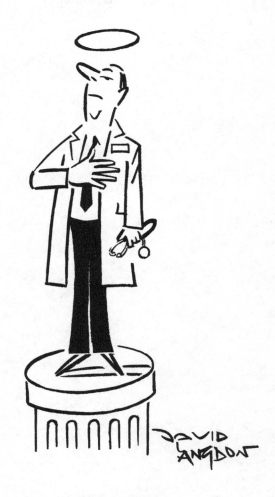

Hippocratic oath

2

Clinical freedom and professional responsibility

Clinical medicine is a personal relationship between doctor and patient; community medicine a more distant link between doctor and population. All walks of medicine involve teamwork between doctors and other health workers. Doctors providing support services also play a full part in these relationships, which rely on complete commitment to the best interests of patients and on absolute trustworthiness.

Trust and honesty

Trust is fundamental: trust that the doctor will not abuse the diplomatic privilege to come and go in other people's lives, to invade their privacy and to have great influence on their decisions. Trust that the doctor will listen carefully, sympathetically and confidentially, will examine thoroughly, will investigate appropriately and as safely as possible, and will advise dispassionately. Trust when a fee is to be paid that the fee will be appropriate.

Truthfulness is as necessary a quality for medical students as for doctors. Perfection is for the angels but it is essential to report and document findings and interim diagnoses accurately, to commit oneself and to learn from having to refine and refine again, to admit when things have gone wrong, to advise candidly without considerations of personal gain and to defer to more expert advice readily when appropriate. Honesty is qualified, not killed, by

13

kindness. It is essential to tell the truth but not always kind to tell the patient the whole truth at once (and who in any case knows the whole truth with certainty?). Patients on the whole prefer a confident and decisive doctor, a definite to a discursive approach. Yet 'doctor's orders' is an outdated concept, useful only as an explanation for patients to pass on to others to justify the constraints their condition imposes on them. More often than not initial diagnosis, investigation and even treatment rests on a balance of probabilities. Explanation and advice need to be tailor-made for each person and situation, explaining as much as is known for sure, as can be understood and is helpful. It is neither kind nor sensible to burden a patient with speculations; it is always right to leave hope and a plan of action however dark the clouds on the horizon seem to be. Risks of a course of action including surgery, or none, must be explained.

The right balance in all situations is hard to achieve. Experience and natural flair both help but there is still more to learn. One's best is not always good enough:

> Far older than the precept 'the truth, the whole truth and nothing but the truth', is another that originates within our profession . . . 'do no harm'. You can do harm by the process that is quaintly called 'telling the truth'. You can do harm by lying. In your relationships with your patients you will inevitably do much harm, and this will by no means be confined to your strictly medical blunders. It will arise also from what you say and what you fail to say. But try to do as little harm as possible, not only in treatment with drugs, or with the knife, but also in treatment with words, with the expression of your sentiments and emotions. Try at all times to act upon the patient so as to modify his sentiments to his own advantage, and remember, to this end, nothing is more effective than arousing in him the belief that you are concerned whole-heartedly and exclusively in his welfare.[8]

Clinical freedom

Students whose course of instruction may have been dogmatic and who may sadly not have learned to question and read around the subject may be surprised and unsettled to discover when they qualify that doctors may with good reasons differ substantially in their diagnoses. More often, and with perhaps less logic, treatments differ. Sometimes it is quaintness or reaction of old age, sometimes the uncritical enthusiasm of youth; at other times it is simply that the evidence is open to different interpretations and conclusions, that the cautious wisdom of those who have seen innovations come and go over the years questions the practical importance of statistically significant but small differences in outcome, especially when set against increased cost and hazard.

Doctors have a responsibility to be as sure as they can be of the diagnoses they make and the effectiveness of the treatment they prescribe. As knowledge increases through the use of controlled trials of treatment and the introduction of continuous audit of clinical practice there is diminishing justification for idiosyncratic approaches or for the use of expensive remedy if the balance of evidence is that a simpler (and often safer) one will do as well. On the other hand, there is a continuing need for flexibility and individual judgement. The traditional and hotly defended concept of clinical freedom is only a legitimate right if fully informed and taking account of the needs of others. Freedom to treat if you are wrong, risky or unnecessary extravagant, is unacceptable. As Professor A. C. Dornhorst once said, 'error has no rights'. In these days, in which fashion tends to be both more dangerous and more expensive, there is force in Hampton's provocative statement that

Clinical freedom is dead, and no one need regret its passing. Clinical freedom was the right – some seemed to believe the divine right – of doctors to do whatever in their opinion was best for their patients. In the days when investigation was non-existent and treatment as harmless as it was ineffective the doctor's opinion was all their was, but now opinion is not good enough.

Clinical freedom died accidentally crushed between the rising cost of new forms of investigation and treatment and the financial limits inevitable in an economy which cannot expand indefinitely. Clinical freedom should, however, have been strangled long ago, for at best it was a cloak for ignorance and at the worst an excuse for quackery. Clinical freedom was a myth that prevented true advance. We must

welcome its demise, and seize the opportunities now laid out
before us.[9]

This is not to deny the ethical duty of doctors to claim the best
possible treatment and care for their patients. It is to accept,
firstly, that because it is possible to treat, it is not necessarily either
kind or constructive to do so. Second, if only marginally justifiable to treat, compromise has to be reached between the technically feasible and the economically justifiable; as Hampton puts
it, where resources are limited 'one man's provision is another
man's deprivation'. Should society invest, for example, in organ
transplants for the few or in hernia and hip operations for the
many, in improved rehabilitation for those who have suffered
strokes, in preventive medicine – or even in improved education
and housing? Eventually these decisions which start as ethical
ones end as political ones.

Ethical dilemmas

Scientific and economic feasibility are only two aspects of the
ethical dilemma. Much can be done but how to decide when it is
ethically correct to do it? Often it is not clear on humanitarian or,
for some, on religious grounds whether treatment, simple or
heroic (the patient being the hero) is right at all.

Ethical views are in ferment: yesterday's truth may be tomorrow's folly; occasionally yesterday's folly becomes tomorrow's
truth. New questions are continuously being raised by rapid
developments in medical science: for example contraception has
become both safer than pregnancy and, in terms of world population, responsible; it has also become inexpensive by Western
standards. But is contraception right, even for Roman Catholics,
or is it wrong? Alternatively, is it sometimes right, for example
only when pregnancy would be a serious threat to the health of the
mother?

The dilemma of when to intervene in illness has also become
much sharper now that treatment for so many conditions has
become more effective and resuscitation more likely to be successful. When Arthur Hugh Clough wrote 'Thou shalt not kill but
thou needst not strive officiously to keep alive', treatment of
pneumonia in a person riddled with cancer or a disorientated

demented person unable to look after himself would have been most unlikely to have altered the outcome. Antibiotics and intravenous fluids might well now prolong the agony for patient, relatives or both and indeed the cost of care in a Health Service desperate to channel its resources to greatest need. Is it right? Action or inaction must be decided case by case taking account of the patient's wishes and all the circumstances.

Only the arrogant or bigoted will claim absolute, universal truth in many of these matters; differences of opinion, responsibly held and in good faith, are inevitable. Differences must be accepted but they must as far as is possible be set out logically and clearly so that they may be examined and re-examined with the changing wisdom of the years. Albert the Great, Bishop of Regensburg is quoted as saying

> One must respect the continued variability of the real and
> not attempt to locate all human actions under one and the
> same universal rule. The real must not be bent to the rule; it is
> the rule which must be adapted to the real.[10]

Law is not a sufficiently sensitive or flexible instrument for guiding the ethics of medical practice, because there is wide and legitimate disagreement on many ethical issues, technical advances make new procedures possible and ethical attitudes change. Lord Devlin advised that the appropriate question to ask the law in these circumstances is

> 'How much authority is necessary?' not 'How much liberty
> is to be conceded' ... that authority should be a grant, and
> liberty not a privilege is the mark of a free society.

Within this freedom different conclusions will be drawn and different, even conflicting courses of action will be pursued; all valid at the current state of wisdom.

Who then should make these agonising decisions on the borders of individual conscience and professional ethics; a committee, the patient, the relatives, the doctor? Although in some countries committees of citizens are charged with some of these decisions, there is no evidence that committees are wiser than individuals. Many of these decisions can be made by the patient, who is entitled to choose whether to be resuscitated or not, but is not entitled to demand and receive euthanasia. In an acute crisis,

however, the patient's wishes are often not known and he may be
unable to communicate or to comprehend. Close relatives should
be kept fully informed and involved in life or death situations but
families cannot always be contacted and they by no means always
agree amongst themselves. Often they willingly leave the final
decision to the doctor, on whom the American College of Physicians has firmly laid the final responsibility for decisions on
resuscitation.

> A decision not to attempt resuscitation is the ultimate re-
> sponsibility of the physician. Such responsibility cannot be
> taken over morally or legally by institutional committees on
> ethics or any other person or group of persons who may be
> available for advice.[11]

Sir Raymond Hoffenberg, while President of the Royal College of
Physicians of London, also argued that the doctor, in close liaison
with the family, was the person to take the final responsibility, not
because of any prior right of the doctor to act as God, but because
only the doctor was in full possession of all the medical facts and,
unlike the family, could act with the detachment essential in such
agonising situations:

> My concern to preserve the central role of the doctor in
> clinical decisions, moral or otherwise, is not a reflection of
> professional self-interest or a wish to perpetuate pro-
> fessional sovereignty. It is based on my belief that such
> decisions must rest on a proper knowledge of all the medical
> consequences of each option, physical and psychological,
> qualitative as well as quantitative; but they must be made
> with critical and professional detachment; and that they
> should be conveyed to and discussed with the patient and the
> family with compassion and with sensitivity.[12]

The final decision of this sort is never easy. It is not taken lightly
and it is difficult to forget. The Revd Dr Davis McCaughey,
churchman, academic, Governor of the State of Victoria and
medical ethicist, insisted that –

> Ethical decisions must be made by those who have to live
> with the consequences of their actions. Hence the import-
> ance of professional ethics, of a tradition, convention, code

to which those adhere who have to take the responsibility for their actions.[10]

In short, the buck stops with the doctor. It will normally be many years before the recent graduate is faced personally with these decisions but from an early stage he or she will have to implement such decisions, sometimes, perhaps, when he does not agree with them, but with a right and responsibility to be involved in making them.

Hippocratic oath

The personal and public ethical responsibilities of doctors converge on these major issues. The Hippocratic oath no longer provides a sufficient basis for professional responsibility. Even modernised versions (Table 2.1) confer an outdated image. Concepts such as dutiful 'respect and gratitude' to teachers, the 'honour and noble traditions of the medical profession' and the 'brotherhood', while worthy and desirable must be earned not

Table 2.1. Declaration of Geneva (1948; amended 1968)

At the time of being admitted as a member of the medical profession:

I will solemnly pledge myself to consecrate my life to the service of humanity;
I will give to my teachers the respect and gratitude which is their due;
I will practise my profession with conscience and dignity;
The Health of my patient will be my first consideration;
I will respect the secrets which are confided in me, even after the patient has died;
I will maintain by all the means in my power the honour and the noble traditions of the medical professions;
My colleagues will be my brothers;
I will not permit considerations of religion, nationality, race, party politics or social standing to intervene between my duty and my patient;
I will maintain the utmost respect for human life from its beginning even under threat and I will not use my medical knowledge contrary to the laws of humanity.
I will oppose all activity which threatens indiscriminate or mass destruction of mankind.
I make these promises solemnly, freely and upon my honour.

demanded. The remaining ideals are unexceptional but where
high ethical standards are both expected and respected by the
public and insisted upon by the profession from the outset of
medical training, a public statement of the Hippocratic oath
seems contrived and redundant. If in fact students graduate (some
would say are even *admitted* to medical school) without the
integrity and dedication necessary for serving in the medical
profession, no amount of recitation of pledges is likely to have a
lasting effect on either their attitudes or their behaviour. Dr
Davies McCaughey has criticised the Hippocratic oath as a
formal basis for medical ethics not on these grounds but on its
paternalism and limited vision:

> Probity, decorum, etiquette, kindness are all important, but
> they are scarcely adequate faced by the puzzling ethical
> issues of our day. Significantly they speak of the behaviour of
> doctors in relative isolation from the needs and wishes of
> their patients; and they have assumed on the part of patients
> a relation of almost complete trust and dependence which
> can no longer be taken for granted.[10]

Even if doctors were absolutely certain in their diagnoses and
correct in their treatments in a patient's best interest regardless of
the doctor's personal religious beliefs, this would of itself be
insufficient reason for *imposing* a course of action. Partly, perhaps, as a result of better general awareness of illness and the
hazards of treatment, and partly because of a general but com-
paratively recent political emancipation which expects government by consent, there is a much clearer, if tacit, recognition that

> the doctor does not inherit his authority or obtain it simply
> by virtue of his training, background or expert knowledge;
> he holds that authority by the consent of his patients.[10]

That being so, there is no excuse for this and many other reasons
for the arrogance sometimes displayed by both young and old
members of the medical profession and even by medical students.
Doctors need to act with the consent of patients, a consent
which must on specific issues be 'informed' consent. Informed in
two senses; first, as is now well accepted, with the patient being
helped to understand the risks of treatment and the risks of no
treatment; second, in a not so widely accepted way, with the

doctor taking the trouble to become fully conversant with the full background and circumstances of the patient, a duty which Lord Scarman has expressed thus:

> not only to advise as to medical treatment but also to provide his patient with the information needed to consider and balance the medical advantages, and risks alongside other relevant matters, such as, for example, his family business or social responsibilities of which the doctor may be only partially, if at all, informed.[13]

Social responsibility and the National Health Service

It could be argued that the doctor's public ethical duty extends further afield because health and effective treatment of disease depends not only on medical science but also on social and economic conditions. For example, for every death of a person of professional or executive status there are two deaths amongst unskilled or manual workers. The incidence of accidents amongst the latter group is three times higher and of mental disease five times higher than the former. Whether doctors are so exercised by the need to secure treatment for indigent patients or to improve their poor living conditions which make it difficult to promote health or consolidate recovery from disease, that they feel compelled to add a political dimension to their professional responsibility is a personal matter. In the UK doctors have the immense privilege of working in the National Health Service (NHS) which, despite its shortcomings, has been overwhelmingly successful in providing treatment regardless of individual ability to pay.

It was in 1944 that the impending birth of the NHS was announced by Sir John Hawton in these words:

> The government have announced that they intend to establish a comprehensive Health Service for everybody in this country. They want to ensure that in future every man, woman and child can rely on getting all the advice, treatment and care which they may need in matters of personal health; that what they will get will be the best medicine and other facilities available; that their getting them shall not depend on whether they can pay for them, or on any factor irrelevant

to the real need – the real need being to bring the country's
full resources to bear upon reducing ill-health and promoting good health for all its citizens.

This revolutionary ideal has succeeded brilliantly, if not perfectly,
for 40 years. Small wonder that the medical profession, the public
and most politicians of all parties give very high priority to
preserving and improving the NHS. This is a jewel in the crown of
Britain as a civilised society, the defence, promotion and evolution of which is the responsibility of the whole population, not
just of the medical profession itself.

Table 2.2. Categories of professional misconduct[14]

Neglect or disregard by doctors of their professional responsibilities to
patients for their care and treatment.

Abuse of professional privileges or skills.

Personal behaviour; conduct derogatory to the reputation of the medical
profession.

Self-promotion, canvassing and related professional offences.

Standards of education and practice – the General Medical Council

Standards of medical education, professional practice and professional conduct are a statutory responsibility in the UK of the
General Medical Council (GMC) with which all doctors become
provisionally registered on graduation at a UK university (or on
passing a nonuniversity diploma) and fully registered on satisfactory completion of the preregistration house officer year. The
GMC has the right, which it exercises from time to time, to inspect
all such 'qualifying' examinations and to require changes in them.
Likewise it lays down guidelines for both the house officer year
and for subsequent postgraduate training.

Professional misconduct in the eyes of the GMC normally falls
into one of four categories (Table 2.2). Professional responsibilities to patients for their care and treatment include those listed
in Table 2.3.

Table 2.3. Professional responsibilities of doctors to patients[14]

'Conscientious assessment of the history, symptoms and signs of a patient's condition.

Sufficiently thorough professional attention, examination and, where necessary, diagnostic investigation.

Competent and considerate professional management.

Appropriate and prompt action upon evidence suggesting the existence of a condition requiring urgent medical intervention.

Readiness, where the circumstances so warrant, to consult appropriate professional colleagues.'

Abuse of professional privileges applies both to privileges conferred by law and those conferred by custom. The prescription of drugs is subject to statutory regulations and these must be observed, including the prescription of drugs only in the course of *bona fide* treatment and not to satisfy addiction either in the doctor or others. Medical certificates must be strictly accurate. Termination of pregnancy must accord with the law.

The trust essential to a proper personal relationship between doctor and patient has already been mentioned. In particular a doctor may only in very special circumstances disclose information obtained in confidence from or about a patient, must not put any pressure on a patient to the doctor's personal financial advantage and a doctor must not enter into

an emotional or sexual relationship with a patient (or with a member of a patient's family) which disrupts that patient's family life or otherwise damages, or causes distress to the patient or his or her family.

On personal behaviour, the GMC is faced from time to time with the need to institute disciplinary proceedings on the grounds of personal misuse or abuse of alcohol or other drugs, dishonest, indecent or violent behaviour. Likewise, although the rules may change, doctors are still prevented from self-promotion, advertising and competitive activity directed against colleagues. They are also expected not to disparage the skill, knowledge, qualifications

Table 2.4. Circumstances in which professional confidence may
legitimately be disclosed[14]

1. With the written and valid consent of the patient or his legal adviser.
2. In the course of shared care with other doctors, nurses and other members of health professions, but making it clear to them that the information is in strict confidence.
3. In particular circumstances, in confidence, to a close relative, this can be a most difficult issue with regard to a professional confidence with a person under the age of 16, without knowledge of a parent. In the words of the 'Advice'

   The doctor must particularly have in mind the need to foster and maintain parental responsibility and family stability. Before offering advice or treatment the doctor should satisfy himself, after careful assessment, that the child has sufficient maturity and understanding to appreciate what is involved ... If the doctor is satisfied of the child's maturity and ability to understand ... he must nevertheless seek to persuade the child to involve a parent, or another person in *loco parentis* ... If the child nevertheless refuses to allow a patient or other such person to be told, the doctor must decide; in the patient's best medical interests, whether or not to offer advice or treatment. He should however respect the rules of professional confidentiality ... if the doctor is not so satisfied, he may decide to disclose the information learned from the consultation; but if he does so he should inform the patient accordingly, and his judgement concerning disclosure must always reflect both the patient's best medical interests and the trust the patient places in the doctor.

4. If in the doctor's opinion disclosure to a third party other than a relative would be in the best interests of the patient, it is the doctor's duty to make every reasonable effort to persuade the patient ... If the patient still refuses, then only in exceptional cases should the doctor feel entitled to disregard this refusal.
5. In response to a statutory obligation, such as notification of an infectious disease.
6. If directed to disclose information by a judge or other presiding officer of a court before whom he is appearing to give evidence ... or to a coroner or his nominated representative to the extent necessary to enable the coroner to determine whether an inquest should be held.
7. Rarely, on the grounds that it is in the public interest, for example when investigations by the police of a grave or very serious crime might override the doctor's duty to maintain his patient's confidence.
8. If necessary, for the purpose of a medical research project which has been approved by a recognised ethical committee.

or services of other doctors. On the other hand, doctors also have the duty, perhaps too reluctantly performed, of informing an appropriate body when the behaviour of a professional colleague raises questions of serious professional misconduct or physical or mental illness.

Fitness to practise is a very difficult issue which is handled initially by senior colleagues, 'wise men', appointed by their peers, and considered eventually by the Health Committee of the GMC. The procedure is designed to be as dignified and fair as it can be. When the Health Committee after due assessment concludes that a doctor's fitness to practise is seriously impaired it may impose conditions on his registration for up to 3 years, or suspend registration for up to 12 months, with regular reviews thereafter. Doctors in these circumstances are encouraged to take early retirement on health grounds.

Perhaps the most difficult ethical area of all for the doctor in a personal capacity is the matter of professional confidence. Circumstances where exceptions to the rule may be permitted, as outlined by the GMC in their *Advice*, include a number of situations listed in Table 2.4.

Professional confidentiality

The GMC's guidance on professional confidentiality makes it clear that where a doctor discloses confidential information he must always be prepared to justify his actions if called upon to do so. A grey area remains in relation to whether a doctor may properly initiate action or only respond to a request. This issue has recently arisen over physical or sexual abuse of children. Both the BMA and the Medical Defence Societies have taken the view that in these circumstances the interests of the child are paramount and the GMC has stated that not only is it permissible for the doctor to disclose information to a third party but it is his duty to do so.

Clearly professional confidentiality is not absolute: it is a fine balance between the wishes of an individual and what is in fact in his best interest; between the rights of an individual, for example to infect others and the rights of others not to be infected, at least unknowingly; between the good of children and the rights of their

parents; and between the right, if any, of a violent criminal to be
shielded from the consequences of his actions when seeking medical assistance. A previous Health Service Commissioner (Ombudsman), Sir Cecil Clothier, commented on this issue in his *Rock
Carling* monograph of 1988:[8]

> One perceives a strange tendency towards absolutism in a
> field where pragmatism is plainly more appropriate. For
> there are obviously many situations in which a doctor may
> find his moral and social duty overwhelmingly in favour of
> disclosure rather than concealment ...
> To declare that an absolute duty of confidence arises merely
> from the relationship existing between the casualty officer of
> the day and a man seeking treatment for a gunshot wound on
> a single day, seems to me to fly in the face of common sense as
> well as to disregard a social duty.
> Moreover, the extent to which doctors are willing to give
> non-medical persons, or medically qualified people having
> no relationship with the patient, ready access to case notes
> makes a nonsense of the absolutist position ...
> The law's view of the matter is, I suggest, admirably practi-
> cal. The technical language of the law groups these problems
> of disclosure of confidence under the heading of 'Privilege',
> that is to say, a law or right which is private or special to a
> person or a situation. One of these privileges is the right to
> keep hidden, or sometimes to disclose without penalty, facts
> which might help the discovery of truth. The fundamental
> rule is that justice is so important to everyone in the orderly
> resolution of the conflicts which arise in society, that its
> interests are paramount and that no information should,
> therefore, be kept from a court of law.
> The only absolute and unqualified privilege against disclo-
> sure of confidential, oral and written exchanges is legal
> professional privilege, that is to say, the right of lawyers to
> keep from a court all oral or written matter which has passed
> between them and their clients in connection with the liti-
> gation ... the judicial process as we know it in this country
> would be impossible without such a privilege.

It is not the purpose of this book to give detailed advice on these
and other ethical issues, only to flag up some of the major issues

about which most of us were hardly aware as students. When faced with an ethical dilemma it is essential to take advice from senior colleagues, a Medical Defence Society, the BMA or even from the GMC itself.

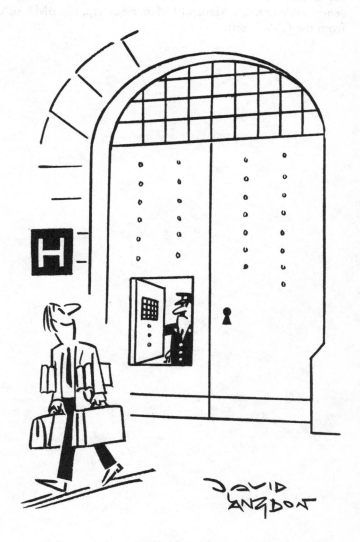

. . . like leaving prison . . .

3

The end of the beginning: 'finals' and the preregistration year

To pass 'Finals' – the final, clinical sections of the Bachelor of Medicine and Surgery degree examinations (MB, BS or equivalent) – is the great goal, the passport to practice which will open all doors. Passing the degree examinations (or an equivalent nonuniversity qualifying diploma) in fact only confers the right to provisional registration with the GMC. The real passport to practice is full registration, effected a year later on satisfactory completion of supervised experience as a preregistration house officer.

Working for the Final MB

After passing the second MB (or its equivalent at Oxbridge and at universities with a more integrated curriculum) during two or three years of preclinical study, the avalanche of information and pressure of learning gives way to the calmer days of the first two years of the clinical course. Calmer that is with respect to academic pressures: psychologically the encounter with patients, their illnesses and their often agonising circumstances is more challenging and disturbing.

Some universities provide an early and gradual introduction to patients while teaching basic medical sciences. Elsewhere, the students, relieved but still somewhat shellshocked from their preclinical course, find themselves abruptly thrown into the clinical water at the deep end, left after rudimentary instruction to sink or swim. Almost all learn to swim, some sooner and better than others but a few never satisfactorily come to terms with patients.

Patients are not only ill, often desperately and mortally ill, but they come from much more diverse backgrounds than most medical students. Patients are, however, only part of a clinical student's rite of passage. Another is the doctors who teach them, who sometimes display nineteenth century arrogance without nineteenth century grace and a view of women worthy, if worthy it be, of the suffragette era. It takes time (especially for mature students) to acclimatise, to accept that times change slowly, that professions change by evolution not revolution and that their teachers, old fashioned though they may be in some of their attitudes are almost invariably committed and will respond warmly to signs of enthusiasm and interest.

Two years of clinical study quickly pass. Gradually the horizon clouds; the future seems less assured. The mountain of information to be brought together in the last year before Finals assumes gargantuan proportions. Realisation dawns that the need to know is driven by the responsibility to do. Clinical responsibility with all its physical, mental and social pressures is just around the corner. Medicine is about to become a way of life, a far more demanding and constraining way of life than had ever been imagined. Accepted, it is deeply satisfying and rewarding; resented, it is a mess if not a disaster.

It pays to start working for Finals from the first day of the clinical course, to adopt an attitude of mind that carefully and critically checks off the necessary clinical skills as they are acquired, to develop a habit of practising them assiduously and to read around each condition as it is seen, keeping personal notes of patients seen as pegs on which to hang each condition. Notes about each condition should be brief, clear, even diagramatic to form a handy aide memoire when revising for Finals in due course. Clinical students are expected to be sufficiently interested, intelligent and intellectually mature to organise much of their own studies for themselves.

The Final MB examination

Universities vary in their approach to Finals; one at least relies on in-course assessment for all except the weakest students. Of the remainder, some space out the clinicals in different subjects over a number of months while others, the majority, end the course with a short burst of written papers, clinical examinations and orals in medicine (including not only general medicine but also child health, psychiatry, community medicine and general practice), surgery (including not only general surgery but also orthopaedics, ophthalmology and ENT), obstetrics and gynaecology and clinical pharmacology (written papers and orals only). Some schools combine the clinicals in medicine and surgery, a sensible step both philosophically and organisationally. Universities which group clinical subjects together for the Final examinations require all subjects to be taken together at first attempt even if they permit failed subjects to be taken singly thereafter. The reason is partly because disease knows no tidy subject boundaries and it therefore makes sense to have a wide background understanding of interlinking and overlapping areas, and partly because it is necessary to demonstrate integration of knowledge in this way rather than to take, pass and forget individual subjects serially.

The written examinations, some of which may be in multiple choice format, require the same discipline and careful strategy as any other examinations. It is so sad as this late stage of university education to see applicants failing because they have not carefully read and reread the questions, have not complied with the instructions at the head of the paper, or have failed to divide the time appropriately between questions. Answers must be legible and examiners have a right to expect university students of five or six years standing to be literate.

Practice and experience are the key to the necessary skill and confidence to pass clinical examinations; there are few short cuts. Examiners can quickly see who has learned to relate well to patients (including the very young, the old and the psychiatrically disturbed), to take well focused histories and to examine thoroughly, effectively and with confidence in the physical signs. They can quickly identify those who are able to synthesise the whole picture into possible diagnoses in order of likelihood, to institute a sensible scheme of investigation and embark on overall management – a far wider process than treatment.

Oral examinations may be more of an ordeal to self-critical students keenly aware of the inevitable gaps in their knowledge than to many of their less perceptive colleagues. On the other hand, no one expects you to know everything and good examiners will concentrate on what you do know and not on the gaps. Oral examinations are more likely to be concerned with understanding mechanisms of disease, with diagnostic awareness and a sensible approach to prevention and management, than with encyclopaedic knowledge.

Although by the time of Finals students are older, more experienced and on the whole wiser than at the second MB stage, most of them find the stress of bringing together all their clinical knowledge and skills for a concentrated succession of examinations very formidable. Systematic preparation by practising clinical skills and personal note-making over the whole of the three clinical years takes away much of the agony. It is always worth remembering that Finals are designed primarily to certify an individual as able to relate well to patients and their families, as sufficiently knowledgeable and sensible to be safe to practise under supervision, and sufficiently receptive in attitude and intelligence to continue to self-educate and re-educate throughout professional life. Candidates pass unless their poor performance or lack of confidence persuades the examiners that they would not safely cope with clinical responsibility. About 90% of candidates pass at first attempt; a small proportion obtain honours in one or more subjects.

Failing the MB

Almost anybody can be sufficiently unlucky with the chance of clinical cases or, occasionally, with a clash of personality with the examiners, to fail Finals once. Failure in one or even more parts is by no means the end of the world and by itself has little if any lasting effect on any career. The Final MB BS can only be taken at intervals of six months but it is permissable meanwhile to sit for one or more of the non-university qualifying diplomas, of which there are three: the 'conjoint', LRCP, MRCS mounted jointly by the Royal College of Physicians of London and the Royal College of Surgeons of England; the Scottish 'triple', mounted jointly by the Royal College of Physicians and the Royal College of Surgeons of Edinburgh and the Royal College of Physicians and Surgeons of Glasgow; and the LMSSA diploma of the Society of Apothecaries of London. Candidates who fail once or even twice are normally not a serious problem either to themselves, their future colleagues or their patients; the issue of those who fail repeatedly and exhaust their permitted number of attempts at university Finals is another matter (see p. 1).

First steps after passing the Final MB

Finals have long been a stressful challenge. In 1841, *Punch* serialised in its first volume the experiences of an apocryphal medical student, Joseph Muff, and his friends. As Finals drew near a remarkable change was noticed:

> a complete transformation, but in an inverse entomological progression – changing from butterfly into chrysalis. He is seldom seen at the hospitals, dividing the whole of his time between the 'grinder' and his lodgings; taking innumerable notes at one place, and endeavouring to decipher them at the other. Those who have called on him at this trying period have found him in an old shooting-jacket and slippers, seated at a table, and surrounded by every book that was ever written upon every medical subject that was ever discussed, all of which he appears to be reading at once – with little pieces of paper strewn all over the room covered with strange hieroglyphics and extraordinary diagrams of chemical decompositions. His brain is just as full of temporary information as a bad egg is of sulphuretted hydrogen; and it is a fortunate provision of nature that the dura mater is of a tough fibrous texture – were it not for this safeguard, the whole mass would undoubtedly go off at once like a too-tightly jammed rocket...[15]

The Final examinations themselves were an event which not even *Punch* could find funny:

We will not follow his examination; nobody was ever able to
see the least joke in it; and therefore it is unfitted for our
columns. We can but state that after having been puzzled,
bullied, 'caught', quibbled with and abused . . . his good
genius prevails and he is told that he may retire . . . he has
passed . . .[16]

Once the initial glow of success has faded and the first few friends
and acquaintances (even the Bank Manager, with intent) has
called you 'doctor', there are three essential matters to attend to
and at least one other to think carefully about. The first is to pay
the fee for provisional registration with the GMC, which licences
the 'preregistration' house officer. The second is to join (for a
much larger fee) one of the three medical defence societies (the
Medical Defence Union, the Medical Protection Society or the
Medical and Dental Defence Society of Scotland). The third thing
to do is to have a really good holiday before taking up the first
house officer post in a few weeks time.

Medical defence societies

The medical defence societies are mutual, nonprofitmaking
organisations set up to provide professional liability insurance
and a wide range of advice to their members on ethical, legal or
contractual issues arising out of their work. They are excellent
organisations which provide a personal and very readily available
service when medico-legal problems arise. More than this, they
fulfil an important educational role in drawing attention to pitfalls in practice, particularly in accident and emergency departments. Insurance companies are beginning to enter the
professional liability insurance field but it is most unlikely that
they will be able to offer such a personal and available service as
that currently provided by doctors for doctors through the medical defence societies.

The cost of subscriptions has rocketed in the last few years
because of soaring legal costs and damages but the impact on
doctors in full time service in the NHS (or in univeristy service
with an honorary clinical contract) has been cushioned by two
recent decisions. Initially, that Health Authorities should reim-
burse two-thirds of the cost of subscriptions of doctors only in

NHS practice, and more recently that the NHS should provide professional liability protection for all NHS doctors. It seems likely that doctors would still be wise to be members of a medical defence society for general professional legal advice but the cost of subscriptions for this limited service should be greatly reduced.

The British Medical Association

It is sensible also to join the British Medical Association (BMA). The BMA negotiates with the health departments, provides evidence to the Doctors' and Dentists' Pay Review Body, makes public pronouncements in the name of the profession on all major issues affecting health or the provision of health care and publishes the *British Medical Journal* (BMJ), which is included in the membership subscription. In addition, the BMA offers many personal services to members; local branches organise clinical meetings and social occasions. While the BMA has in the past tended to be very conservative in its policies, it has recently taken a much more forward-looking view on many issues including controversial ethical issues, the form and function of the NHS, career structure in the NHS and the importance of university-based undergraduate medical education. Most doctors join the BMA but some prefer more radical organisations such as the Medical Practitioners Union (MPU) or, as consultants, the Hospital Consultants and Specialists Association (HCSA). The Medical Women's Federation exists to improve the position of women in medicine.

Superannuation

A superannuation scheme has to be chosen at this stage. a recent change in legislation has given members of occupational pension schemes the right to opt out in favour of personal pensions arranged by commercial insurance companies. At present there is no reason to believe that any alternative scheme is preferable to the NHS superannuation scheme and there seems to be very good reason to join the NHS scheme.

Preregistration house officer posts

Most UK medical schools have their own pool of house officer posts open to their own graduates. A number of students prefer to make their own arrangements at hospitals near their homes, or at which they have worked, or where they happen to know a consultant for whom they would like to work. Posts available to UK graduates normally exceed the number of graduates by about 10%, so there is no need to worry about not being able to find a post. Postgraduate subdeans normally handle the matter and will advise. The time for application varies from scheme to scheme, some allocating more than a year before qualification, others only a few months before. Perhaps the most important point to remember when applying for posts in a scheme, if not constrained in choices by marriage, friends, or dependent relatives, is, after stating preferences, to leave the possibilities as widely open as possible in order to have the best chance of getting a post. If intending to specialise in a hospital specialty there is much to be said for obtaining at least one house officer post in your university hospital. If intending to go into general practice it is wise to look for a house officer post in an area of the country in which you would like to find a vocational training scheme and to settle subsequently.

Preregistration house officer posts became compulsory about 40 years ago. Previously, most newly qualified doctors went straight into general practice. For about 20 years after house officer posts became compulsory most general practitioners only undertook the minimum two posts before going into practice but since then all doctors have had to undergo a period of at least three years further training for general practice and more for other specialties. When it was normal to go into practice after one year as a houseman the practical training and experience provided by the undergraduate course had to be as comprehensive as possible, much more so than is either necessary or appropriate today. Now, whatever specialty a doctor is destined to enter, a substantial period of further training is required and both the undergraduate course and the house officer year have a much more general educational role in providing what the GMC terms 'basic medical training', a foundation of attitudes, understanding and experience relevant to any specialisation.

The role of house officers

GMC regulations require that the twelve months of house officer posts include at least four months in Medicine and four in Surgery 'in the widest sense'. The norm is six months in each, of which at least three in each involve experience of general acute emergencies, and the other three may be in more specialised posts. Four months in general practice in a health centre is permitted and the few schemes which offer this option are popular; the intention is to give experience of the circumstances and role of general practice to those planning to stay in hospital specialties, rather than to start training general practitioners.

House officers must reside in hospital both to be readily available and to obtain full educational benefit by living 'over the shop'. Life 'on the House' used to be part of the life experience of house jobs, including membership of a lively young working men and women's club, which in my personal situation had the imposing address 'Number One Knightsbridge'. Food was cooked for the residents in 'the cottage', not in distant hospital kitchens. Bacon and eggs were always left out in the kitchen at night for any who had missed supper or were working late into the night; unhealthy food perhaps, but we felt valued. Few of us were married and married accommodation was unheard of. The wife of a colleague was rather disconcerted when at 7 o'clock one morning after an uncomfortable night sharing her husband's single bed, the maid knocked at the door, looked in, and called out 'cup of tea, nurse?'. Now, for whatever the many reasons, few house officers live in except when on-call; food is institutional, surroundings are sad and camaraderie is little more than a flash of goodwill at Christmas.

Housemen have both administrative and clinical tasks. The administrative role is to ensure good communication and organisation within the whole team, with the patients and their relatives (including explanation and reassurance) and with the referring general practitioners, besides keeping the notes and collating the results of investigations. The clinical role is with the registrar or SHO to provide emergency diagnosis (including negotiation of urgent investigations with already hard-pressed diagnostic departments), initial treatment and planning of the next steps. Symptomatic relief day by day (and night by night), performance of standard practical procedures and follow-up investigations are, in the first instance, the house officer's responsibility. New graduates are usually relatively ill-equipped to cope well with symptomatic relief of relatively minor symptoms of pain, nausea, constipation, anxiety and reactive depression, unless they have taken the trouble to follow carefully patients they have clerked, or have carried out student assistantships or shadow house officer attachments. But control of symptoms of relatively minor import- ance to overall progress can make all the difference to comfort and peace of mind.

Keeping patients' records

Housemen must keep concise, legible and accurate notes from day to day, including all positive findings, important negative find- ings, daily follow-up notes, a record of who has been told what about the patient's illness and a list in the margin day by day of tests ordered to record what was requested and when. Also it is good practice to keep a cumulative flow chart of the results of all laboratory investigations, so that the pattern and trends can be seen at a glance and unexpected findings noticed.

The amalgam of technical, pastoral and managerial roles of the house officer under careful supervision provide the experience and help to develop the skills listed in Table 3.1.

Communication with patients, relatives and colleagues

Maintaining good communication is an essential part of the job. First, it helps in hospital to weld a team out of doctors, nurses, paramedical staff, social workers, administrators, porters and all others who contribute to the patients' care. Second, it is excellent practice and common courtesy to telephone the general prac- titioner when a patient dies, is about to leave hospital or, indeed, to give a progress report or to obtain additional background information. It is not always possible to get through and attempt- ing to do so may be very time-consuming but it is important to try. In any event a short *pro-forma* summary must always either be taken away by the patient or put in the post on the day of

Table 3.1. Objectives of the preregistration house officer year [17]

To understand the nature and implications of, and to make an appropriate initial decision about, each problem presented to him as a doctor.

To plan and carry out, under appropriate supervision, the investigation, treatment or management of and rehabilitation after acute and chronic illness, and to participate in programmes for promotion of good health.

To apply knowledge of science and of logical method to the assessment of clinical problems and to continue to develop the ability to assess the reliability of evidence.

To develop knowledge and understanding of disease processes.

To maintain attitudes appropriate to the practice of medicine, which include respect for the dignity of the patient and concern for the relatives, awareness of the legal and ethical aspects of medical practice, together with appreciation of the importance and implications of professional confidentiality.

To be aware of the limitations of his or her own knowledge and skills and to be ready to seek help.

To continue to develop the capacities for self-education and self-audit.

To learn effective and economic use of laboratory and other diagnostic and therapeutic services.

To learn safe practice in relation to radiation protection, blood products, body fluids and tissues in the ward and laboratory, and to have regard at all times to the safety of patients and health care workers.

To gain experience in teaching others, effective teamwork, the management and administrative aspects of medical practice and the work of these bodies which plan, advise and assist with the organisation and provision of health care in the community and in hospital.

discharge. It is most important to see that the general practitioner's name and address is in the notes so that the final summary can be sent to the right place and person. Thirdly, patients and their relatives must be kept informed about the nature of the illness and its progress, their fears and worries answered as best as can be and the right balance struck between optimism and reality in looking to the future. Supporting the dying can be a harrowing experience for which no amount of theoretical instruction adequately prepares, important though instruction is. With the help of senior colleagues this skill has to be learned on the job.

Sir Cecil Clothier has recently drawn attention to one particularly accident prone aspect of hospital life which rapid and sympathetic communication can do much to defuse, namely last minute cancellation of operations:

the patient prepares himself to meet with dignity and cheer-
fulness an event of which he may be, despite his denial,
mortally afraid. At the least he will be conscious of an
occasion which calls for courage and composure. As the
patient reaches the crest of this wave of preparatory effort, it
is quite commonly and casually announced to him that his
name has been taken off the list.[8]

Even with the best management, postponements cannot be
entirely prevented but explanation and reassurance are very important if anxiety and disappointment are not to turn into anger.

Sir Cecil Clothier also gave advice about the importance of
talking and listening to relatives, a task sometimes overlooked,
not least because relatives often visit when the houseman is either
off duty or busy on-call.

Talking to relatives of the sick is laborious, exacting and
time-consuming … But it is as much the delivery of health
care as the prescribing of medication. For this, as in so many
aspects of human communication, listening is probably
more important than talking.

Even with the best, sooner or later a case will go wrong, usually
because of an unfortunate combination of circumstances – ill
luck, not negligence. Medical defence societies are understandably very cautious about any admissions of error because of
possible legal consequences and it is essential to take your defence
society's advice in each individual situation in consultation with
the consultant for whom you are working. It is also essential to
document honestly, precisely and continuously what has
happened, what steps you have taken to correct it and what
information you have given and to whom. Nevertheless, wherever
possible, openness has much to recommend it. Sir Cyril Clothier's
advice from the health ombudsman's seat was 'It pays to apolo-
gise. Nothing disarms a critic more completely or quickly than an
admission of error'.

Stresses and strains

For most doctors the preregistration year is in many ways the
hardest of their lives. The stress of making decisions for the first

time, of giving bad news to patients and their relatives and of working through a stream of interruptions can be greatly eased by understanding and helpful nursing staff, the more experienced of the junior medical staff and by consultants who have not fogotten the bewilderment and tiredness of being a houseman. More senior resident help should always be available for advice but they have many other tasks and need their sleep too. The worst feature is lack of sleep and interrupted sleep, many of the calls being for minor symptomatic, technical or administrative problems, many of which the nursing staff could and would cope with if they were allowed as much responsibility as they are in other countries, for example in adjusting intravenous infusions and administering drugs through them.

A one-in-three rota of resident duty first or second on-call is currently the norm, amounting to an average weekly commitment of 83 hours. A regular commitment greater than this is unacceptable. Some rotas are less demanding. The contract includes a few more hours if the regular daily programme formally begins before nine and ends after five. Contracts also often include a commitment to cover for colleagues during periods of holiday, sickness or study leave either because locums are simply not available or satisfactory or because of very high locum agency rates which health authorities are unwilling to pay.

These long hours continue for several years as a junior doctor in hospital. Others are now in the front line of interruptions but personal responsibility for more complicated technical procedures and emergency decisions increases. In some SHO posts, such as neonatal paediatrics, the combination of long hours and ceaseless, intricate technical demands in emotionally draining situations is worse than in any preregistration or more senior posts, but usually being an SHO is more congenial than being a houseman. In addition to the demands of the work the surroundings are usually depressing – accommodation spartan and food both poor and not available at the odd moments when there is time to eat.

All these demands add up to a job which at this stage is very different from students' perceptions of their future career, summed up in North American experience as follows:

Patient care is an insistently demanding experience. The house officer is crucially dependent on machines and technological approaches. For many young doctors, such an emphasis makes being a physician highly impersonal, and for almost all, makes it far less pleasant than they ever imagined...

The tempo is intense. Interns and residents only rarely sit back, relax and talk at length among themselves about their patients, and certainly almost never can they do so with patients.

Discussions at bedside rounds address life-saving treatments and not the character of the lives of the patients. House officers are developing greater expertise in how to do procedures and to use technological means but are learning less about how to talk to patients so as to understand their lives as well as their illnesses.[18]

Prospects for improved working conditions

Does it really have to be as hard as this? Are improvements in sight? Clearly the specialties differ in the nature of their work but the situation described accurately represents acute medical and surgical services, including paediatrics and obstetrics. The current situation is not acceptable but there are many aspects to the problem, none of which can immediately be resolved without cutting service or imposing a radical change in consultants' contracts. All the difficulties can be overcome given time, firm purpose and money.

Several solutions to the problem of excessive hours worked by junior doctors are possible and all are likely to be needed to some extent. More junior doctors is not an option. Already there are too many junior staff for the career posts available, a situation which *Achieving a Balance* has set out to remedy over the next 10 years (see p. 4). A substantial decrease in registrars, a moderate reduction in senior registrars and an increase in consultant posts is planned. Recent medical manpower predictions indicate that at least the current number of medical students is required to meet future needs. If fewer can become registrars in the most popular specialties many will either spend longer in SHO posts (which if posts are increased in number will reduce hours) or become better distributed across specialties.

Better use of existing staff by greater crosscover between related specialties has some mileage but although specialties may seem to require similar skills they may in fact demand very different experience. Clinical audit had shown, for example, that emergency vascular surgery has a far better outcome performed by vascular surgeons than by general surgeons. A full share of resident emergency duties by all grades of junior medical staff, including senior registrars (who are not fully incorporated into resident duties in all centres) would also help.

With governmental and, quite understandably, public pressure for a more consultant-led service the days draw nearer when consultants, who do not normally have any *resident* on-call duties but are available to advise at short notice and short distance, may be required to assume some of the resident duties of registrar/ senior registrar, duties which all consultants on appointment felt with relief that they had left behind. The problem is not simply one of altering attitudes, life styles and contracts, nor is it simply one of money (although a change of contract would doubtless be expensive in terms of time off in lieu if not in additional sessional payments). Consultants often have duties in more than one hospital, far apart in some country districts, and outpatient clinics at several locations, quite apart from the demand for domicilary consultations at general practitioners' requests. They also have administrative responsibilities around their health districts and perhaps further afield. Far-reaching changes in their wider responsibilities and way of life would be needed for them adequately to provide the continuity of more senior support currently provided for preregistration house officers by registrars and senior registrars.

In many hospitals SHOs already provide much of the intermediate cover for preregistration house officers. Not all SHOs, however, have sufficient experience to provide adequate intermediate cover, even with consultants maintaining as close an involvement as possible.

Another solution is to concentrate acute emergency services on fewer sites. To an extent this has happened already in response to

economic pressures. But in country districts there are limits to
which services can safely be concentrated, and in all districts
public opinion is strongly behind local hospitals serving local
needs. Political pressures will ensure that progress in adopting this
solution will be slow and limited.

As a temporary expedient it would at least help to make junior
doctors feel valued if long hours were recompensed by overtime
rates of pay increasing with hours of duty. Double the current
overtime rate has recently been introduced for hours above 96 per
week. Clearly this is only a temporary expedient because it does
nothing to reduce tiredness or strain. Legislation on maximum
hours has so far been regarded as too inflexible. Change will come
and future generations of junior doctors can only get a better deal.
At the end of their training they will, however, if specialising in a
hospital specialty find a rather different style of consultant post.
Some conflict during training seems inevitable, between the need
to gain practical experience and the need to find time and energy
to prepare for higher examinations and indeed just to keep up
with developments.

Full registration with the GMC

The sensation on leaving hospital at the end of the preregistration
year is like leaving prison. There is one more cheque to pay to
achieve full registration with the GMC and it is then time to start
rising from the ranks. Perhaps with *Punch*'s Joseph Muff there is a
temptation to look back

> upon student revelries with an occasional return of old feel-
> ings, not unmixed, however, with a passing reflection upon
> the lamentable inefficiency of the present course of medical
> education pursued in our schools and hospitals, to fit a man
> for medical practice.

Inefficient the course may still be 147 years later, and imperfect its
orientation for today's and certainly for tomorrow's world, but
almost all the products of the system rise magnificently through
all the demands and pressures to the challenge and opportunity of
the preregistration house officer year, emerging tired, fulfilled and

much wiser. All that now remains to be done is to submit to the GMC, with cheque, your completed certificates of satisfactory completion of two preregistration house officer posts for full registration to be granted.

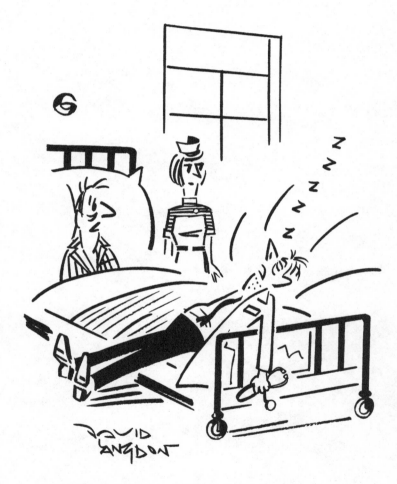

'I happened to mention I wasn't sleeping too well...'

4

Setting the sights: basic training programmes and professional qualifications

Basic specialist training (general professional training)

Basic specialist training, as the GMC describes this period, or general professional training as the Royal Commission on Medical Education 1965–68 (The Todd Report) put it, are much the same thing. All are agreed that general experience and training is appropriate before specialisation but there are wide differences between specialties as to the desirable length of this period. It is partly a moment for consolidation of knowledge, widening of experience and acquisition of general practical skills, and partly a time of career decision-making. Some graduates are so sure of their career intentions that they move as fast as they can into narrow specialist posts and plough that same furrow until they reach consultant status by the shortest possible route. Others are just as sure but prefer to move towards their chosen goal through a process of wider education and experience. Most, perhaps, are not sufficiently firm in their career intentions to be able to narrow them down precisely and welcome the opportunity to sample different specialties to help their career intentions to crystallise.

The GMC recommends that basic specialist training

occupies two or three years following full registration, during which a doctor acquires increased but supervised responsibility for patient care, and develops the wide range

47

of general and basic specialist skills needed for practice in the
specialty concerned.

This period of training is normally undertaken in the senior house
office grade.

The Joint Committee on Higher Medical Training (JCHMT)
sees the purpose more widely still, emphasising the importance of
being able to retain an option of changing direction and therefore
of remaining pluri-potential for as long as possible. As specialisms
become increasingly narrow it surely becomes ever more important to have a wide base of knowledge and experience before
committing oneself to a particular specialty for the rest of one's
life; not only has disease a knack of presenting as a wolf in sheep's
clothing to an inappropriate specialist, but communication with
colleagues (and not only about patients) is so much easier with
knowledge and experience of what they do. It is refreshing therefore to read that the JCHMT sees the aim of the period of general
professional training to be 'to enable the trainee to obtain broad
medical experience and to identify the specialty which he/she
hopes ultimately to follow', and encouraging to see that periods of
up to six months in general practice, community medicine, pathology, psychiatry, surgery or obstetrics and gynaecology would
be recognised as acceptable parts of the background to general
(internal) medicine, accident and emergency would surely also be
not only acceptable but desirable. While for most other specialties
an early move into posts in that specialty is encouraged, the
JCHMT recommends that for medicine (which includes a large
number of sub-specialties – see Chapter 8) not more than one year
should be spent at this stage in posts exclusively confined to
general medicine and not more than six months in any other post
confined to a single specialty.

Surgical and especially pathology specialties diverge at an earlier stage of postgraduate training than do most others but there is
a wide range of opinion and practice about the amount of *basic*
training – uncommitted to any specialty but directed at acquiring
general skills – that should be obtained before entering a
specialty. In surgery, experience up to the level required for the
present Part II fellowship or just beyond is generally taken as
appropriate before entry to a subspecialty although subspecialisation in ophthalmology, ear, nose and throat and plastic surgery

often starts at SHO level. It could be argued that this lack of more general experience is unduly narrowing. As with undertaking research, it is essential to find out what is the usual pattern for your desired specialty.

Application for SHO posts

For most graduates, applying for a senior house officer post at the end of the preregistration year is the first experience of applying for work outside the sheltered world of their own medical school, the first formal face-to-face encounter with an interviewing panel since their successful application to medical school. Interestingly, no one questions the appropriateness of interviews in appointments to posts in medicine or other professions, although many question the value of interviews at entry to professional training when those same qualities of commitment, humanity and communication which matter so much in the teamwork of providing a service are already discernible. How it is that subjective assessment of these essentially unmeasurable qualities is generally accepted at age 24 but selectively rejected at age 18? Perhaps it is argued that there is a difference between selection for a particular post and entry to a multidimensional profession?

Both the job application and interview merit careful preparation and presentation. It is not difficult, even in current competition, to obtain an SHO post, but it may be difficult to get the particular post which, where and when you wish. Your application should be typed unless you have beautiful copper-plate writing. Amazingly, applicants still submit scrappy, illegible applications; why spoil chances from the start? The application should look good (not fussy) and should clearly state the bare bones of academic and professional record together with a trimming of seductive flesh – those achievements, distinctions and experiences which make you not only different but more attractive than the others. Profession of undying allegiance to each specialty you wish to sample is neither necessary nor desirable; much better to be honest and simply to indicate how the post fits into the pattern of your proposed postgraduate training as you see it at present. Everyone knows that realistic aspirations take time to shape and that circumstances modify appetite.

It is often difficult to know at what stage of the application
process to visit a hospital and the consultants for whom you
would work if successful. While there are general rules of eti-
quette there are also substantial differences of opinion. Canvassing is not permissable but where does a legitimate 'casing of the
joint' end and canvassing begin? If short-listed for a post at any
level it is sensible and acceptable from all points of view to inspect
both post and prospective colleagues and to be inspected in
return. It is rightly death to an applicant's chances to appear at
interview without having visited the hospital and at least asked to
meet the consultants concerned. Who can be considered a serious
applicant who has not studied the job and assessed by asking
relevant questions whether the team is one into which he or she
would fit? While it is important to find out sufficient about the
post and people to motivate application, it is probably normally
neither necessary nor desirable to do more before the short-list is
known, at least at junior level. If in doubt, a diplomatic call to the
consultant's secretary with an offer to visit before short-listing but
asking for advice cannot go amiss.

Look respectable at interview but not over-dressed; it both
shows respect to the interviewers and indicates that however great
a rebel you may be at heart you are prepared to be a presentable
number of a professional team. Speak clearly, look at the person
you are addressing, be honest yet diplomatic. Listen carefully to
questions, look for their point and go carefully but straight to it. It
is normally a mistake to apply for a post, to accept an invitation to
formal interview and then to refuse the post. Problems can and
should be explored and resolved beforehand and not at interview.
Occasionally it is necessary to raise formally at interview constraints which will determine whether or not it would be feasible
for you to accept the post. They should, however, have been
raised beforehand and be mentioned now only for formal recognition and perhaps for formal assurance that the problems will be
resolved.

Common characteristics and objectives of SHO posts

Although SHO posts generate a large number of applications,
90% of preregistration house officers obtain their first SHO post

within two months of first application. The nature of the work in all the acute specialties is similar to that of the preregistration posts but with more responsibility for decisions and procedures, involvement in outpatient work in clinics and in the Accident and Emergency Department, a shared responsibility with the registrar or senior registrar (if there is one) for inpatient summaries and, usually, less form-filling and routine continuity work than a preregistration house officer. SHOs straddle, in different porportions in different posts,the tasks and responsibilities of preregistration house officers and registrars.

Whatever the specialty, the SHO has the opportunity to develop practical skills associated with it. Surgical SHOs will begin to learn and to undertake under supervision common surgical operations and a wide variety of practical techniques. Likewise in medicine, techniques such as gastrointestinal endoscopy and cardiac pacing are part of the specialty commitments. There is opportunity too to perfect techniques learned but perhaps not often practised as a preregistration house officer, such as cardiac resuscitation, lumbar puncture, chest drainage and peritoneal dialysis. Medicine in its widest sense is still a very practical art and procedures which not long ago were looked upon as highly specialised and dangerous have become commonplace, not least because the technology of the equipment involved has advanced.

Responsibilities in outpatients or in accident and emergency should always be undertaken with a senior colleague readily at hand for advice. Discussion of cases at the time is important for many reasons including medico-legal considerations. Systematic joint review by consultant and junior staff of patients attending outpatient clinics is necessary to prevent the cumulative accretion of outpatients who readily become addicted to hospital visits but would be more appropriately and personally followed by their general practitioners than by a succession of junior doctors.

Dictating short, to-the-point summaries of inpatients is an extremely important link in the chain of communication between hospital and general practitioner. There are few good excuses for failing to get formal summaries despatched within a week of a patient's discharge. Hospital administrators have an absolute responsibility to provide the necessary secretarial support, while doctors have no less a responsibility to confine the summary to the absolute minimum of information needed for its purpose of com-

munication. Inpatient summaries should neither be complete records of every finding and investigation, nor research documents.
All the essential information should be in the day to day notes,
legible and well ordered. The amount taken from that larder and
served up on the summary plate can normally be very small
indeed.

Delays in summaries reaching general practitioners are one of
the simplest, commonest and most reprehensible failings of the
hospital service. If all backlogs were slashed by a one-off tranche
of two-line summaries, if all new summaries were of half the
previous average, if administrators were rapidly taken to task if
the delay in sending out summaries exceeded one week because of
secretarial insufficiency and all immediately responsible doctors
were reprimanded if the delay was due to their tardiness or
verbosity, the quality of communication in the hospital service
would be transformed overnight. The use of word processors may
of course soon become so much a part of every medical student's
and doctor's life that doctors, like journalists, may quickly come
to generate their own copy for the permanent record.

During this formative period of general professional training
doctors in all specialties will ideally develop the foundation of the
formidable list of attributes set out by the GMC (Appendix 1).
The fact of the matter is, however, that with one in three for
general emergency duties and/or for providing special investigations, such as cardiac pacing or emergency endoscopy, together
with an increasing need to prepare for specialist examinations,
many SHOs and registrars feel resentful and even desperate at the
demands of a treadmill which seriously disrupts their homelife
and leaves them too tired to properly do all they have and want to
do. Much but not all of the on-call duties at this stage still require
living-in at hospital.

Preregistration house officers accept their intensive duty in the
flush of enthusiasm of having qualified at last and of learning so
much so quickly. At the SHO level the learning curve is not so
steep, the demands of examinations begin again, future prospects
seem uncertain and unsettling, and domestic ties increase. Forty-
four percent of doctors marry within two years of graduation; a
further 22% were already married by the time they qualified.[3]

In specialties without acute intaking responsibilities the
demands are much less intense: these include medical specialties

such as dermatology, oncology, neurology, rheumatology and genito-urinary medicine (sexually transmitted diseases) and pathology specialties such as haematology, immunology, histopathology and microbiology.

Most surgical specialties have responsibility for emergencies. Acute work is also an inevitable part of the task of SHOs in obstetrics and gynaecology. Accident and Emergency departments clearly have to provide a 24-hour service but at least the duties are structured into a formal shift system which other SHO posts are not; night and weekend duties in other specialties are an addition not an alternative to regular working hours.

Most doctors during the general professional training stage have an idea of the broad category of work they wish to undertake. This is sufficient to indicate the higher professional diploma which should be aspired to and worked for alongside all the day to day demands of providing a service. The relationship between general professional and higher specialist training is introduced here and summarised in Appendix 2.

Medical specialties

Membership of the Royal Colleges of Physicians (MRCP(UK)) is the first goal for those aiming at a medical specialty and also for many of those thinking of general practice, psychiatry or pathology (especially haematology), and even for a few of those planning a surgical career but aware of the great value to a surgeon of a good basic training in medicine. Part 1 of the examination is common to all medical specialties whereas Part 2 can be taken either in general medicine or in paediatrics.

Part 1 of the MRCP(UK), is entirely theoretical although based on clinical practice; it tests knowledge of a wide range of medical conditions and the underlying medical science. It can be taken 18 months after graduation but it is a waste of money and may delay subsequent attempts if taken without sufficient preparation. Part 2, which is written, clinical and oral, can first be taken 12 months after Part 1 and after at least one year of responsibility for acute medical emergencies in either adults or children. The crunch for most candidates is the clinical, in which a high standard of clinical skill and common sense based on experience is required. A pass or borderline mark must be obtained in the written section before proceeding to the oral and clinical sections. Candidates who then fail the clinical and oral section may not carry forward a pass in the written section of Part 2 but have to sit the whole of Part 2 again.

The written section of Part 2 falls into three parts: case histories, data interpretation and projected material. The case histories are designed to test ability in diagnosis, planning of investigations and management. The data interpretation involves the results of different types of investigation. The projected material includes photographs of patients, radiographs and pathological material about which questions of diagnosis, investigation and treatment are asked.

The clinical examination is similar in approach to the MB Finals but requires a higher standard of clinical skill, a standard no higher, however, than the small number of students winning honours in medicine in the MB have already achieved as students. One hour is allowed for a long case followed by 20 minutes during which a pair of examiners check with the candidate on the accuracy of history and physical signs obtained and probe understanding of the significance of both in relation to diagnosis, investigation and management, including aftercare. Thirty minutes is spent seeing short cases in the presence of another pair of examiners, each examiner leading for approximately half the time. The purpose is to test the candidate's ability to elicit quickly and confidently physical signs related to disease in all the major body systems. The short cases are probably the most discriminating test of clinical diagnostic ability and quickly sort out the good diagnosticians from the not so good, but at the borderline there is always an element of luck and gamesmanship.

The oral examination lasts 20 minutes and is conducted by a third pair of examiners, so that each candidate is examined in the course of clinicals and orals by six different examiners. This examination tests understanding of basic principles, including applied physiology, capacity to deal with clinical situations, including emergencies, devising plans of management of given situations including preventive medicine and public health.

Altogether, the MRCP(UK) is a formidable examination which requires wide knowledge, confidence in clinical skills and good clinical common sense. It cannot be passed simply on book knowledge. About one-third of candidates pass each time, few at first attempt. The examination is held simultaneously in Edinburgh, Glasgow and London and their associated centres in provincial hospitals for the clinical examinations. Examiners are exchanged between the three Royal Colleges to ensure equal standards. Candidates can choose either of the three main centres. The number of attempts at the MRCP(UK) is currently limited to a maximum of four at Part 1 and six at Part 2 although there is a proposal to permit three attempts at Part 2 at each of the three centres. Without the MRCP there is effectively no prospect of a career in a hospital medical specialty. Courses for the examination help many to pass, not least by giving them some uninterrupted study time away from work, but a number of good doctors simply do not have the examination technique or *sang froid*; others are not sufficiently well organised in their approach. That is not to say that they cannot make a great success of a different specialty; many do.

Surgical specialties

Those who want to become surgeons have two parallel and to some extent interacting paths to run. First they must now get onto a training programme with a 'numbered post' which indicates that the job is recognised for surgical training with the objective of a consultant post in the United Kingdom. Second they must obtain the appropriate professional qualifications which include a fellowship of a Royal college, (FRCS) taken presently in two parts and often a higher university degree (MS, MD or PhD – desirable, see below). Currently both sets of requirements are under review and are passing through a period of rapid change so that the description and advice found here is, of necessity, interim.

Training programmes

The common practice has been for surgeons of nearly every intending type to pass from their preregistration jobs to an SHO in either a specialty such as cardiothoracic, orthopaedic or urological or to a post in accident and emergency (A & E) as both

are a necessary requirement for the Part 2 fellowship. A & E posts
in particular are attractive because their regular hours of work
provide an opportunity to study for the Part 1 fellowship. There
are a slowly growing number of posts which combine A & E with
a demonstratorship in a basic medical sciences department
(usually anatomy) and this enhances the chances of a candidate
being successful early in the Part 1. Alternatively a *fulltime*
(though poorly paid) demonstratorship can be taken in an Anatomy Department for up to a year. Such a post may be intellectually
gratifying but is a relatively slow way to the Part 1.

Having got the Part 1 out of the way, further experience is
sought at SHO/registrar level in both general surgery and a
specialty, depending on what has been done before the Part 1, so
as to complete the requirements for the Part 2. Orthopaedics is a
common choice, not least because posts are numerous and also
orthopaedic patients are relatively easy for examiners to acquire
for the clinical in Part 2. Such experience can be obtained either by
moving from job to job on an *ad hoc* basis or by becoming part of
a pre- or transfellowship rotating programme. The latter is preferred but understandably there is a great deal of competition for
such organised rotations.

All this training, while necessary for the diploma of fellowship,
is not at the moment a guarantee that the individual will proceed,
but the situation may soon change. It is only when a postfellowship registrar becomes a senior registrar in his chosen specialty
that he is given a 'numbered post' which implies that he is going
on to 'higher' – as distinct from 'basic' – surgical training to
become a consultant. It is not surprising that there is intense
competition for places in higher surgical training and the registrar–senior registrar bottleneck has plagued the surgical side of
the NHS since the service began. An attempt is now being made to
open up this stricture by numbering registrar posts so that, given
the necessary qualifications, a trainee will pass as a numbered
person through post-fellowship registrar to senior registrar and
eventually consultant in a continuous and predictable way. It is
obvious that these posts will be fewer than those presently available so that the effect will be to push the bottleneck back into the
SHO–registrar transition. Numbering of registrar posts in general
surgery is expected to be complete by the end of 1989 and it is only
these posts (known as Career Registrars) which will then

confer training status. The transition from the old type to the new type registrar will take place over about two years as existing registrars either get posts in higher training or drop off the ladder.

Professional qualifications in surgery

The Part 1 as it is presently designed is entirely an examination in the basic medical sciences. There are multiple choice question papers (and for the English College essays also) in anatomy, physiology/biochemistry and pathology/bacteriology together with an oral examination in each subject. Results in the written part are used in some colleges as a filter to eliminate the oral for candidates who cannot be expected to pass. While there is reciprocity of recognition between the Part 1 examinations of the Royal Colleges of England, Scotland and Ireland, each college still sets and holds separate examinations. To prepare, a candidate will in addition to seeking out the most useful appointments (see above), endeavour to attend a primary fellowship course of varying duration. Some of these – though not necessarily the best – are organised by the Royal Colleges. In that the present Part 1 is something of an artificial exercise candidates are advised first, to take the examination at the earliest possible opportunity while knowledge is still reasonably fresh and also so as to get an irksome hurdle out of the way and, second, to attend a course which much enhances the chance of passing.

Part 2 of the FRCS may not be taken until after the necessary clinical experience in general surgery, orthopaedics, A & E and specialist surgery has been obtained and three years have passed from full registration. The examination comprises written papers and orals on the general principles of surgical care, operative surgery and surgical pathology. There is both a clinical and an oral examination. Obtaining the FRCS allows the surgeon to proceed to 'postfellowship' appointments which give further experience and can ultimately lead to the higher surgical training already discussed. It is thus currently an 'intermediate' examination (in general surgery) though many overseas graduates who obtain it return to their own countries and set up in independent surgical practice. The Part 2 FRCS in ophthalmology and otolaryngology (ENT) are already taken later and function as 'exit' examinations.

Plans are well developed – and will probably be implemented in 1992 at the latest – to change the Fellowship examination structure. Part 1 will become a two part examination in basic science and in the principles of surgical care and of surgery in general (not to be confused with 'general surgery' which is now to become a specialty in its own right). The new Part 1 will be taken perhaps a little before the present second part and should then be a condition of entry into one of the new style numbered registrar posts. There will then be an 'exit' examination in the specialty of the registrar/senior registrar's choice at about the fourth to fifth year of professional training. This examination will probably contain basic science relevant to that specialty and will be a necessity for 'accreditation' (see Chapter 8).

Obstetrics and gynaecology

For obstetrics and gynaecology, Membership of the Royal College of Obstetricians and Gynaecologists (MRCOG) is normally essential before proceeding to higher specialist training, whether or not the FRCS (or even the MRCP) is also obtained. The exception is that both the Royal College of Surgeons of Edinburgh and the Royal College of Physicians and Surgeons of Glasgow provide a Fellowship examination in obstetrics and gynaecology, which a few offer as an alternative to the MRCOG; most of those who take the FRCS in this specialty, however, offer it as an extra and not as a substitute for the MRCOG. The Part 1 of the FRCS in obstetrics and gynaecology is as for the other surgical specialties and the written paper and oral examination on the Principles of Surgical Care is the same as for general surgery. The remaining written paper, clinical and oral is specific to obstetrics and gynaecology.

The MRCOG examination is also divided into two parts. The first is a multiple choice examination in the basic medical sciences related particularly to obstetrics and gynaecology and can be taken after full registration with the GMC. The second part is, like the FRCS, an intermediate examination which can only be taken after at least three years in the specialty and must be passed before starting higher training as a senior registrar. Written papers, multiple choice papers, a clinical and oral examination make up Part 2. In addition, candidates are required to submit a volume of case reports and commentaries on which they may be questioned in the oral examination. As of 1988 fewer cases are required in the volume of case commentaries and no short reports but an annual log book recording all obstetric and gynaecological experience is submitted each year by trainees in the specialty until they have passed the MRCOG. Five attempts only are allowed at Part 1 and they must be made within a period of five years from the first attempt. A similar rule applies to Part 2.

Psychiatry

For psychiatry, work needs to start at SHO/registrar stage for Membership of the Royal College of Psychiatrists (MRCPsych) which must also be acquired before continuing to higher specialist training as a senior registrar. A number of students obtain the MRCP(UK) first as evidence of a wide grounding and ability in general medicine; others enter from or on completion of a general practice vocational training scheme.

The MRCPsych examination has just been revised and only the new arrangements are relevant to those now considering a career in psychiatry. This examination is also in two parts. Part 1 is a multiple choice (MCQ) and clinical examination, designed to test clinical skills in assessment. It must be passed within three years of starting full-time, approved psychiatric training, (or an equivalent period of part-time training). The MCQ covers basic psychopathology, methods of clinical assessment in psychiatry, basic clinical psychopharmacology and neuroanatomy, neurophysiology and neuropathology. Part 2 can be taken soon after passing Part 1 provided three years post-registration training in approved posts has been completed, including 12 months in adult general psychiatry. The examination includes multiple choice papers, an essay paper, a short answer paper, a clinical and an oral examination on patient management problems.

One of the two MCQs is devoted to sciences basic to psychiatry and the other to topics on the theory and practice of clinical psychiatry. The short answer and the essay paper cover both aspects but a Research Dissertation may be submitted in place of the essay paper, although this option is seldom exercised. The sciences basic to psychiatry are psychology, neurophysiology, neurochemistry, clinical pharmacology, social studies, genetics, epidemiology and statistics and research methods. The clinical aspects covered in the papers include the assessment and management of psychiatric disorders in all age groups, including both clinical and community aspects, mental handicap, forensic psychiatry, psychotherapy, substance misuse, epidemiology and the history of psychiatry. Up to four attempts are permitted at Part 1 and five attempts at Part 2.

Anaesthetics

Intending anaesthetists need to work for the Fellowship of the Faculty of Anaesthetists of the Royal College of Surgeons (FFARCS), all or most of the examinations for which, have to be passed before entering higher training. Some begin by passing the MRCP(UK) as witness to their competence in general medicine.

Examination for the FFARCS is in three parts. The first may be taken as soon as full or limited registration with the GMC has been granted and covers the principles of anaesthesia in all common specialties including anaesthetic aspects of the management of acute medical and surgical emergencies. A basic knowledge of relevant aspects of physiology, pharmacology, physics, anatomy, medicine and surgery is also required. There is an MCQ, written paper and two orals. The objective of the examination is to identify

> a level of performance which will distinguish a safe practitioner, able to handle any emergency without unnecessary further deterioration for a limited time until more experienced or skilled help can be obtained, and one who understands the extent of his abilities and the circumstances in which assistance needs to be sought.

Part 2 may not be taken until Part 1 has been passed. The examination tests knowledge of relevant basic science in physiology and pharmacology in detail (including relevant physics and statistics) by a multiple choice paper and two orals.

The third Part, like the FRCS and MRCOG, is an intermediate examination. Applicants must have been qualified for at least four years and have substantial experience in the specialty. The examination covers general principles of anaesthesia and analgesia as well as anaesthesia in special branches of surgery. Intensive care, clinical medicine and surgery, clinical chemistry and applied physiology and pharmacology all form part of the knowledge and experience tested.

Diagnostic radiology

Specialisation in radiology may begin one year after full registration. The first examination to be passed is Part 1 of the Fellowship of the Royal College of Radiologists (FRCR). Not more than four attempts at the examination are permitted. Many entrants to radiology first acquire the MRCP and a few the FRCS. The final examination may not be taken until three years have been spent in approved posts; it consists of two multiple choice question papers, two clinico-radiological oral examinations and a film reporting session.

Radiotherapy and oncology

Radiotherapy and oncology also requires a first and final examination. The first part may be taken after one year in an approved post and covers physics, medical statistics, pathology of neoplastic disorders and principles of cancer basic sciences including radiobiology. Four attempts only are permitted. Three years after passing Part 1, Part 2 may be taken. This includes essay and multiple choice papers, an oral, a clinical and a practical examination in radiation treatment planning. The complementary specialty of medical oncology requires the MRCP (see Chapter 4).

Pathology specialties

The pathology specialties have hitherto required medical graduates to have 18 months general laboratory training and experience in pathology (or other approved training) and to have passed the primary examination for Membership of the Royal College of Pathologists (MRCPath) before entering higher training. During the preparation for the primary in recognised departments the candidate was expected to gain experience in at least four of the five disciplines: chemical pathology, haematology, histopathology, immunology and medical microbiology. One subject was offered as special subject and this was examined by a practical and an oral. In addition there was an MCQ which covers the four main branches of pathology together with questions on immunology, statistics and the basic medical sciences. Exemption from the primary examination could be obtained on the basis of membership or fellowship of several of the other Royal Colleges, the Diploma in Clinical Pathology and several MSc examinations but exemptions will not apply to the new examination.

Specialisation will soon begin on entering the chosen branch of pathology and it appears that not only will the wide general training in the different branches no longer be required but wide experience may be difficult to acquire in any formal training scheme. The training period will still be five years. The trainee will still be assessed at the end of that period and the MRCPath awarded at that stage, but the current general primary and specialised final examinations will be replaced by an examination after three years of fulltime approved laboratory training in one specified subject, and an even more specialised examination after a further two years in posts recognised for higher specialist training.

The examination at three years may be taken in chemical pathology, clinical cytogenetics, haematology, histopathology, immunology, medical microbiology, oral histopathology, toxicology or virology. It may also become possible to offer neuropathology and forensic pathology. Two written papers will be set, one probably including a multiple choice section. The practical and oral parts are expected to be similar to the current formidable final examination in which the examination is tailor-made for each individual and lasts at least two days at a hospital where the applicant has not previously worked.

In histopathology, for example it is anticipated that the practical will include performing an autopsy and being questioned on it; surgical histopathology with 15 out of 20 slides to be reported on in three hours; and cytology with 8 out of 10 slides to be reported on in one hour. Candidates will also be expected to present a certificate of technical competence in performing frozen sections and to report on 5 of 6 sections within an hour.

The examination at five years permits a wider range of alternatives than the current final FRCPath. An oral is part of each option. The options are, first, general histopathology with slides and a test including fine needle aspiration and exfoliative cytology; second, a special subject tested as for the general histopathology; third, a thesis on published work. The special subjects include cardiopulmonary, gastrointestinal, renal, paediatric and gynaecological pathology and cytopathology. It is anticipated that the first option will be appropriate for an unspecialised District General Hospital (DGH) post, the second option for a post in a large DGH or academic department which encourages subspecialisation, and the third for a post in an academic department with a large research interest with some opportunity to take part in diagnostic work in the knowledge that support from other senior staff is always available.

Clearly the details of the examinations will differ in the different branches of pathology, especially in haematology which includes a clinical examination.

Community medicine/public health

For community medicine the first part of the Membership of the Faculty of Community Medicine (MFCM) must be passed before entering higher specialist training, while the MFCM itself is almost an exit examination, marking the successful completion of higher specialist training in the subject. Only one further year of training is required after passing the examination before the trainee is ready for a consultant post.

The Part 1 examination for the MFCM consists of three written papers which 'cover the academic basis of community medicine in its broad sense', comprising population (structure, dynamics and health), methods of enquiry (survey and related methods in the health field, statistical analysis of data), factors affecting health (heredity, environmental agents, nutrition), principles of disease control, health, human behaviour and social policy (the individual in society, origins and development of health and social services) and the management of health and social services (the nature of management, organisations management roles and functions, planning and resource allocation, the economist's approach).

The Part 2 is in the form of a written submission and an oral, the written submission being a folio of reports based on the candidate's own practical experience. This part has to be taken within three years of passing Part 1 but it is intended that work for Part 2 starts before Part 1 is passed.

General practice

No additional diplomas are essential for entry to general practice but there are many which mark the acquisition of relevant experience and expertise. Many while taking SHO posts obtain one or more of the following which can normally be acquired on the basis of six months of experience: Diploma in Child Health (DCH), Diploma in Anaesthesia (DA) or the Diploma of the Royal College of Obstetricians and Gynaecologists (DRCOG). Some acquire the MRCP and a few the FRCS before entering general practice. Membership of the Royal College of General Practitioners is not mandatory: it formally tests wide areas of knowledge needed although not all practices regard the qualification as desirable. Three main areas are tested: clinical practice (health and disease, human development, human behaviour), medicine and society (sociology and epidemiology), and the practice (organisation and administration). Written papers include essay and multiple choice papers. An oral examination covers discussion of a log diary prepared by the applicant of 50 consecutive patients seen in a normal working week and a discussion of clinical problems, diagnosis and treatment.

Occupational health

The discipline requires a general understanding of industrial technologies and the measures taken to ensure protection of the health and welfare of people at work. These measures include epidemiological methods of detection and surveillance of occupational diseases and accidents, methods of health surveillance and legislation related to health, safety, and welfare in industry, and systems of compensation for occupational disease. Other aspects include the relationship between health and capacity to work, occupational toxicology, communication skills with workers, management and trades unions, and the structure, organisation and management of occupational health services.

Three years of general professional training including at least six months in occupation medicine is required before sitting the examination for the Associateship of the Faculty of Occupational Medicine (AFOM). The examination consists of clinical, practical and oral parts and submission of a journal. The clinical, examined jointly by general and occupational physicians, consists of one long and some short cases with emphasis on occupational and social factors related to the illness. The practical includes an epidemiological exercise, projected material, radiographs and occupational health findings for comment. The journal is an account of four weeks occupational health practice carried out in the previous 12 months and the oral examination is carried out on this.

Membership of the Faculty of Occupational Medicine (MFOM) is awarded later on the assessment of a thesis, dissertation or published work.

The pressures of general professional training

In summary, all specialties with the exception of general practice require a formidable but attainable higher diploma. Preparation for the chosen qualification demands determination, systematic organisation and the stimulus of a definite goal. Clinical work all too easily fills every hour of the day and much of the night. Tiredness tempts to well-earned relaxation once the clinical pressure is off. But there is still academic work to be done because acquiring a consultant post of your choice depends on passing the necessary diploma as soon as possible. So difficult is it to work sufficiently systematically while on the job that it is important to take full advantage of study leave entitlement (see Appendix 3). By the end of the period of general professional training your career mind should have been made up to the extent that initial steps have been taken on a pathway which leads to the necessary qualifications.

The pressures upon junior doctors from their clinical work, postgraduate examinations and from life itself are enormous. If tempers sometimes fray or manners are abrupt the reason is more likely to reflect those pressures rather than any personal inadequacy or a fundamental failure of the process of undergraduate and postgraduate medical education. Patients may be demanding, unreasonable or simply ill and unaware; doctors may be exhausted. While there are pressures and even faults on both sides I have great sympathy with the doctor who recently wrote to a national newspaper in reply to criticisms of traditional, clinically-based medical education, saying:

> When a junior doctor is confronted with a four-hour clinic on Monday afternoon, having had less than eight hours sleep since Friday morning, and his first patient complains that he has been kept waiting 20 minutes, it is very hard to believe that five years of integrated social science training at medical school will be able to prevent the doctor from behaving in a way which may be interpreted as insensitive[19] . . .

5

Grasping the nettle: final career choice

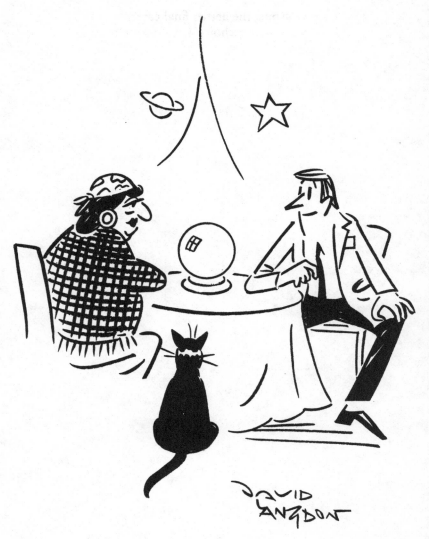

... final career advice ...

5
Grasping the nettle: final career choice

Sooner or later, the die must be cast. Final choice is constrained by many factors, including limited job opportunities, specific domestic commitments or difficulty in passing specialty diploma examinations. Several Royal Colleges or Faculties limit the number of attempts at their specialty examinations, just as universities rightly limit the number of attempts at Finals. It may seem hard that one must pass within the allotted number of attempts or seek a different specialty, but standards are high and competition tough. Not that the ability to pass examinations and standards of practice are necessarily always closely related; but experience suggests that in general they are related and who is to judge the exceptions? High standards are in the public interest and there is a rough, pragmatic justice in selection by first past the post. 'Standards' are not simply a matter of knowledge but of clinical wisdom (which specialty examinations certainly attempt to test) and ability to cope with testing and changing demands.

First choice

Not every doctor can enter the specialty of first choice and many take time to decide what they in fact would like to do. Most start with an imperfect vision of what the different specialties offer, what they as doctors are most suited to, and they possess little information about the balance of national needs. It is not unreasonable that doctors trained, as it were, by public subscription

Table 5.1. First choice of career corrected for ties by doctors who qualified in 1974: changes of mainstream between 1975 and 1981 (Figures are numbers of choices, corrected for ties, rounded to nearest whole number)[20]

Choices in 1975:	Choices in 1981													
	Medicine	Paediatrics	Surgery	Obstetrics and gynaecology	General practice ± other	Psychiatry	Community medicine	Pathology	Anaesthetics	Radiology	Radiotherapy	Other medical	Non-medical	1975 Total (%)
Medicine	146	17	14	2	122	14	3	14	10	12	6	9	–	368(22.0)
Paediatrics	7	38	2	1	48	1	9	1	2	4	2	1	–	114(6.8)
Surgery	11	1	153	2	59	2	2	5	20	4	2	2	1	261(15.6)
Obstetrics and gynaecology	4	1	4	27	19	1	1	3	3	2	2	2	–	65(3.9)
General practice ± other	13	4	7	8	480	20	16	7	18	6	2	4	7	592(35.4)
Psychiatry	1	–	–	–	11	39	3	1	1	–	1	1	1	58(3.5)
Community medicine	–	1	1	–	4	1	4	–	–	–	–	1	1	9(0.5)
Pathology	7	1	2	–	10	1	4	33	2	2	1	1	1	61(3.7)
Anaesthetics	2	1	1	1	16	1	–	1	45	1	–	1	1	70(4.2)
Radiology	2	–	–	1	7	1	–	1	1	9	–	–	–	22(1.3)
Radiotherapy	2	1	–	1	5	2	2	1	1	1	5	1	–	14(0.8)
Other medical	2	1	3	1	14	1	2	1	–	–	1	8	–	32(1.9)
Non-medical	1	–	–	–	2	1	1	–	–	–	–	–	3	6(0.4)
1981 total (%)	197(11.8)	63(3.8)	186(11.1)	43(2.5)	797(47.7)	78(4.7)	42(2.5)	64(3.8)	103(6.2)	38(2.2)	16(1.0)	29(1.7)	15(0.9)	1670(100.0)

Changes of (less than 0.5, including zero changes, are shown by a dash.

should be seen as a national resource to do what is needed. In the words of George Bernard Shaw: 'Up to a certain point doctors, like carpenters and masons, must earn their living doing work the public wants from them'. But in that case the Department of Health should be informing new graduates where the particular needs and therefore opportunities are. Public demand by itself is a poor guide to proper provision and division of service; sections of the population who need most may be those who demand least. Shaw was not necessarily at odds with the BMA, which stated on the eve of the introduction of the National Health Service that: 'Doctors should, like other workers be free to choose the form, place and type of work they prefer without Government or other direction'. It all depends what is meant by 'direction'. The Department of Health has a responsibility to decide where and in what specialties the medical posts in the NHS will be. Doctors must follow opportunities and opportunities should follow needs; encouragement not direction would be appropriate.

Changing aspirations

Changing career choice after the preregistration year, once or even more often, is both reasonable and normal. Parkhouse & Ellin[20] found in a study of 2350 doctors who qualified in the UK in 1974 and were followed for 11 years, that only 31% of those who gave complete replies in two-yearly surveys had retained their original choice of career; 30% had changed once, 30% had changed two or three times and 9% had changed four or five times. Medicine, surgery and paediatrics were the main losers over that period (reflecting limited career opportunity in those oversubscribed specialties) and general practice was the great gainer (increasing from 35 to 48% of first choices). The greatest proportional increase, although absolute numbers were small, was a five-fold increase in community medicine. Gains from one specialty to another can be seen by reading across the columns in Table 5.1 and the losses by reading down the columns.

Parkhouse & Ellin also investigated career intention and its determinants seven years after graduation by combining the returns from 3053 male and 1396 female graduates of 1974 and 1977. Domestic circumstances were most important in the final choice of general practice and community medicine and were overall more important in the career choice of women than men in all specialties except for those entering nonmedical careers. Promotion prospects had encouraged recruitment to less competitive specialties. Self-evaluation of aptitude and ability was an important factor in relation to all choices but especially in psychiatry. Financial circumstances were not of great consequence except with regard to men choosing general practice, 'other medical' and nonmedical careers. Experience as an undergraduate influenced choice of obstetrics and gynaecology and psychiatry but not of general practice, which was the predominant first choice throughout. Teaching in general practice has developed substantially since those cohorts were undergraduates and might now be found to have a more formative role in career decisions.

Limitations of early career advice

Career advice, formal or informal, was found to have little impact. Better and more systematic advice might reduce the initial mismatch between interest and opportunity but this cannot be assumed to be so. Career opportunities in specialties which do not have a high profile in the undergraduate course could, for example, be specifically highlighted. Nothing, however, is likely to replace the need to taste and feel one's way by experience over a number of years. The one factor above all which would encourage appropriate career choice would be a clairvoyant's knowledge of who was to marry and where, when and whom; career choice might be better informed but what a dull world it would be. Less than one-quarter of students are married by the time they qualify. The high statistical chance of marriage within five years of qualification does not in practice persuade house officers to take full account of the impact of probable marriage on their careers. Allen found that:

> Men and women tended to choose specialties or change to another specialty for very similar reasons at this stage of their careers (the pre-registration year), often because they liked or were good at a subject. The realities of life in those specialties seemed to play very little part in their decision-making at these stages, and it appeared that women often

embarked on their careers at registration regarding themselves as doctors first and potential or actual wives and mothers second. Few seemed to foresee the constraints under which they might be conducting their careers, and there was strong evidence that many were over-optimistic or under-informed.[3]

Sydney Smith put it another way: 'As long as boys and girls run about in the dirt and trundle hoops together they are both precisely alike'. At entry to medical school women can be forgiven for not being able to grasp fully the career constraint that gender confers upon them, but five years later it cannot in fact be that they do not know the statistical realities, only that a gulf exists between the individual and the statistics for very understandable reasons. Eventually about 90% of men doctors and almost as many women doctors marry; of those who marry nearly 70% marry within five years of qualification. The tendency to marry during this period may be diminishing, for only 65% of men and 55% of women doctors in their late twenties surveyed by Allen were married or living as married five years after they graduated in 1981. Against the background of this major area of personal uncertainty so important to realistic career choice, advice and counselling may have far less potential than critics of its currently minor role allow. The domestic scene clarifies for most two or three years after registration and can then and only then be taken into account realistically in making a definite career choice. Personality, skill and past experience will already have focused intentions; success or failure in specialist examinations will have sharpened that focus; domestic circumstances now add the finishing touches. The possible avenues are many. While details of the qualifications required have been summarised in Chapter 4 and the nature of the work in each is outlined in subsequent chapters, the principal differences in the nature of the work and its demands in the broad brush of specialties may appropriately be considered here.

General differences between hospital specialties

Medical specialties tend to attract the introvert, reflective (some might say indecisive) and surgical specialties the extrovert, decisive (some might say dogmatic) characters. Exceptions, of course, abound. Surgical specialties do demand greater manual dexterity and decisiveness than most medical specialties, but generally not more than any reasonably dextrous person can develop. Most surgical specialties involve a substantial component of emergency duty for which, during the training years, residence in hospital on-call is necessary. General medicine has similar on-call commitments. There are, however, more medical than surgical subspecialties which do not have a significant out-of-hours component and therefore harmonise more readily with domestic responsibilities. Consultant surgeons, at least those unsupported by senior registrars, have to undertake a large proportion of the emergency surgery themselves, day and night, unpredictable demands which can be very intrusive upon family life. Few women set out to become consultant surgeons, but some do, married or not, and do very well. Consultant general physicians without senior registrars are in a similar position to their surgical colleagues but the nature of the work is more to provide advice than to undertake practical procedures.

Obstetrics and gynaecology has a very substantial out-of-hours commitment. The great attraction of obstetrics is that most patients and their infants are healthy, and that the patients have something very positive to show for their labours. Clearly women, especially those with children, have much to offer in this specialty but the demands are in formidable conflict with a settled domestic life.

In all the acute clinical specialties rapid decisions have to be made. Neither the outcome of intervention nor the consequences of doing nothing are always easy to assess. Surgical decisions are in many respects more obviously far-reaching in their consequences than medical. Most clinical decisions have to be taken on less than complete evidence – a best and carefully considered decision in the light of the available evidence. Those accepting clinical responsibility must develop the ability to weigh evidence and to make and to justify decisions (in court of law if necessary) – sometimes very far-reaching and controversial decisions. To be able to live with the outcome of these decisions, which with hindsight may seem to have been mistaken, errors of commission or omission, is a very important part of a clinician's psychology. It is not as simple today as it was in the sixteenth century when

Francis Quarles wrote to say 'Physicians of all men are most happy; what good success soever they have, the world proclaimeth, and what faults they commit, the earth covereth'.

Psychiatry also has its emergencies but fewer than general medicine, surgery and obstetrics. The specialty attracts divergent thinkers and calls for interest and practical skill in handling disturbed individuals. Psychiatry is a specialty which calls for a broad mind and a calm, pragmatic heart.

Anaesthetists in particular have long insisted that they cannot work safely continuously night and day. They have approached nearer to a shift system of responsibility than other specialties. In addition to sessions in the operating theatre, labour ward and pain relief clinics, anaesthetists routinely examine and assess patients before operation and many have administrative responsibility for running an Intensive Care Unit. Their hours are irregular and include working at night, but with good organisation and support, their responsibilities are predictable and compatible with domestic responsibilities.

Pathology specialties attract doctors of more laboratory and less clinical frame of mind, although a strong element of clinical interest runs through all they do. After the early training phase there is little medical emergency work in these specialties and they therefore have an attraction for those with other responsibilities. On the other side of the coin, there are few extra duty payments and the salary is likely to be less than that of junior doctors in acute clinical specialties. At consultant level the salary is the same as for other consultants. Clinical immunology and, particularly, haematology, are more clinical and bridge pathology and clinical medicine.

Radiology has emergency commitments but since the introduction of gastrointestinal fibre-optic endoscopy which has removed a large proportion of gastroenterological emergencies from their work, the emergency work is largely centred on neurological/neurosurgical and cardiovascular units. Interventional radiology has become very highly skilled, requiring both practical dexterity and ability to relate well to patients. Imaging techniques have in many areas changed the emphasis from conventional radiology to scanning. Radiotherapy is allied to radiology but is in many ways a different discipline, having primarily a therapeutic role.

Specialties outside hospital

All the previous specialties are hospital-based and traditional in form and function. In contrast, general practice, community medicine and community health exploit different dimensions of health care. General practice is concerned with primary health care (in contrast to the 'secondary' referral practice of hospital doctors at the request of general practitioners, and 'tertiary' practice of highly specialised hospital units taking patients from other hospitals). In other words, with care of unstructured ill health, with health education and with preventive medicine in a community setting in which the circumstances rather than specific disease may be responsible for the symptoms. In this context, the general practitioner's knowledge of an individual over many years, and of the family and their social and economic conditions, is often much more relevant to treatment than knowledge of pharmacological therapeutics, although he certainly needs that too.

General practitioners work from a health centre or from a surgery at home. They normally live in the community they serve, spend much time conducting surgeries, less time on home visits by day (and occasionally by night) and they also take an interest in education about health and in personal preventive medicine. Much of the latter, including immunisations, is organised by the practice nurse. Business management is an important framework for the service, the organisational detail of which is often delegated to a practice manager. General practitioners also frequently undertake part-time sessional work, often as clinical assistants in hospital (particularly in medicine, accident and emergency, anaesthesia and psychiatry) or, for example, as a police surgeon, examining people in custody and taking appropriate blood samples. General practice is varied, flexible, based at or near home and suitable for changing commitments over the years. It is a more convenient job for women doctors with domestic commitments than many hospital specialties.

Community medicine, also known as public health, offers yet another approach to health, a global view of health care, health care policy and measurement of the outcome of steps taken to improve the health of whole communities. Doctors are often criticised for concentrating too much on disease in the individual rather than health of the population. Sir Douglas Black has rightly seen here a false antithesis.

> I believe it to be the norm that the interests of the individual and of the population of which he forms a part are congruent, and to that extent an antithesis between individual and population medicine is false.[21]

In a nutshell, he takes the very reasonable view that prevention and treatment are complementary, not alternative. The tools of the job, besides a good background knowledge and experience of clinical medicine and infectious disease, include administrative and management skills and epidemiology. Public health is an expanding discipline likely to be at the heart of future health policy. It offers an exciting challenge, good promotion prospects and compatibility with domestic commitments.

Medicine and marriage

In Allen's survey, two-thirds of women doctors and one-third of men who were or had been married reported that marriage had been a constraint on their careers.[3] More than half of recently qualified medical graduates now marry doctors and many of the remainder have spouses with their own professional careers to fashion. It is often very difficult to find suitable posts for both in the same locality. The frequent moves currently required of doctors in the early years of postgraduate training compound the problem. More rotational training schemes within one hospital or group of hospitals would help. The geographical problems of partners with their separate careers to develop are, of course, by no means restricted to medicine. Bank managers, academics, school teachers, businessmen and women, lawyers, career civil servants and many others have similar problems.

Women have the additional constraint of fitting in pregnancies and running a home, even with husband's help. Men were found in Allen's survey often to be prepared to put a normal family life before specialty or career advancement, but the career consequences of having children almost inevitably fell hardest on the women. For both partners the conflict lies not only in the hours of work, or the need to continue to prepare for examinations, important though both factors are, but also in the absorbing interest of the job. There are some advantages in husband and wife following the same profession. At least they fully understand each other's professional difficulties and enjoy what Medawar referred to as 'the special comradeship of travellers on the same road (one that winds uphill all the way)'. At the same time he cautions anyone from marrying a person too engrossed in his or her career, in his case, as a scientist:

> Men or women who go to the extreme length of marrying scientists should be clearly aware beforehand, instead of learning the hard way later, that their spouses are in the grip of a powerful obsession that is likely to take the first place in their lives outside the home, and probably inside too.[22]

One of the most difficult questions facing married women doctors is whether to start a family before or after completing higher specialist or vocational training (by which time they are well into their thirties). Whatever else, it is essential to complete pre-registration house officer posts. Most women in fact have children while still in training posts. Provided the doctor has been in full-time service in the NHS for at least one year, and provided an undertaking is given to return to work for at least three months afterwards, 18 weeks maternity leave with pay is due, normally beginning 11 weeks before the baby is due, but considerable flexibility is possible.[23]

Women doctors on planned rotations have the right to return to the next planned post after maternity leave. If the contract ends after the eleventh week before the baby is due, the contract will be extended to give the full 18 weeks leave. Many mothers with good family support manage to continue in full-time work with this bare minimum of maternity leave but it is not easy and for many it is impracticable.

Part-time training

A career in an acute specialty in particular can often be combined with responsibility for a young family only through part-time training, which is theoretically available in any training grade, under the provisions of the DHSS scheme PM(79)3 introduced in

1979 to provide part-time training for doctors with domestic responsibilities, physical disability or ill health. Posts must be at least halftime and accreditation takes longer in proportion to the sessions served; emergency duties and on-call commitments are *pro rata*. Below senior registrar level, posts have to be negotiated locally with District or Regional Health Authorities and the new arrangements to be introduced under *Achieving a Balance* have yet to be announced.

For part-time senior registrar posts, a national competition is held centrally each year for a limited number of personal authorisations. The posts are supernumerary but the same credentials are demanded as for full-time posts. Having in this way secured manpower approval the successful doctors have first to construct with local consultants a suitable post which, *inter alia*, must not reduce the quality of the training of other junior staff. Then they must obtain educational recognition of the proposed training post as suitable by the appropriate national Joint Committee on Higher Training (JCHT). Finally they must persuade the local Regional Health Authority to fund the post. The road is long, hard, complicated and bureaucratic. A small amount of part-time training is achieved through opportunistic job-sharing but the strict relationship between training and career posts envisaged under *Achieving a Balance* would seem to discourage job-sharing unless related to established shared consultant posts, which of course, may not be in the right place at the right time for suitable applicants.

Established part-time training posts and consultant posts are currently few and far between but their expansion would seem to offer the best hope of making the best practical use of the increasing number of married women doctors who have much to offer the NHS but also have other responsibilities, which are an essential part of their reasonable aspirations and fulfillment. The practical difficulties over the particular specialties and specific locations are formidable.

Once vocational training for general practice has been completed it is not too difficult to find part-time work as an assistant but to become a principal in general practice is more difficult. General practitioners, it seems, may feel that part-time partners do not pull their weight and cannot provide a desirable level of continuity of care; local Family Practitioner Committees (FPC) may be concerned at the cost implications in terms of practice allowances. Many women working part-time in general practice, on the other hand, strongly believe with justification (as do those in hospital medicine) that they deliver substantially more than their strict sessional commitments.

There are other part-time career opportunities in medicine apart from those in hospital or in general practice. These include community health, working for Health Authorities or Local Authorities in areas such as family planning or child health or working in schools or community clinics. The new Staff Grade, soon to be introduced in the hospital service under *Achieving a Balance*, may also be suitable for part-time service. Of the doctors surveyed by Allen[3] 56% of the women were working fulltime and 36% were working part-time.

Retainer scheme and the need for additional support

If at an early stage a doctor takes time out on account of domestic circumstances and would otherwise be completely unemployed, a DHSS 'retainer' scheme provides for an annual grant of £155 towards the expenses of maintaining registration with the GMC, membership of a medical defence society and a subscription to a professional journal. The doctor is required to attend at least seven educational sessions each year and work at least one half-day a month, but not more than one day per week. The work done cannot be counted towards accredited training. Details of the scheme, which offers a tenuous lifeline to an eventual return to practice can be obtained from Regional Postgraduate Deans or from the personnel departments of Regional Health Authorities.

The ideal solution is to enable married women with children to train and work fulltime. Other countries seem to find ways of achieving this and we surely could learn from them. Better means of delivering domestic support or fiscal measures such as income tax relief to help couples pay for the expensive help they need in order to enable both partners to stay at work seem essential. The problem is political not educational and is not confined to medicine. Nevertheless, Britain is at great risk of wasting the skills of its women doctors and the enormous national investment which has been made in them. In a real world, limitations on the freedom of career choice of married doctors, especially of women doctors, may be inevitable but the limitations need not be as formidable as they currently are.

Academic posts

The demands of posts in all specialties are similar in the nature of their clinical commitments whether held in the NHS or in a university department. University posts provide more opportunity for teaching and research and indeed impose contractural obligations to contribute to the progress of the subject by research. The clinical commitments are generally lighter, if only because the team is usually larger, and so clinical duties can be shared. Lighter clinical duties mean a smaller emergency on-call commitment and this in turn, as in pathology, results in fewer opportunities to supplement basic earnings with extra duty payments.

Clinical academics at consultant level do not enjoy all the rights of NHS consultants. In particular they do not have the opportunity to earn freely from private practice although in several universities clinical academics now have similar privileges to fulltime NHS consultants in this respect (see p. 165). NHS allowances for removal, assistance with mortgages and other practical aspects of moving job and home are more generous than those of the universities. After many years of hard bargaining and uncertainty, clinical academic salaries are linked to NHS fulltime salaries. Clinical academic staff employed by universities but holding honorary contracts with the NHS work as equals with their NHS colleagues, very much part of the team in university hospitals, both in service to patients and in teaching, to which NHS staff make very substantial contributions. Relatively few NHS staff continue to be active in research but some make outstanding contributions there too.

In spite of the remaining financial disadvantages, which are probably inevitable if clinical academics are to apply themselves fully to their academic responsibilities, many doctors find the benefits of more time for teaching and research, the stimulus and satisfaction of both activities, and of being part of an academic community in the university outweighs the material disadvan-

tage. Whether their spouses and families share their view is more
doubtful as they look enviously at the life style of the families of
NHS consultants and general practitioners. Relative to other
academics, however, the clinicians are financially favoured and
deserve to be because of their year-round continuing clinical
responsibility to the NHS.

Other employment for doctors

There are of course, many jobs outside the NHS and universities
in which medical training is either a necessity, such as a medical
adviser in industry, or a doctor in the armed forces, or a bonus,
such as in medical journalism, publishing or the theatre – including Jonathan Miller and Sir James Paget's student in the last
century who became 'well esteemed in gentile comedy'. Most
careers which lack a clinical commitment offer more convenient
and regular hours, quite apart from their different attractions,
and they need be no less interesting or demanding. 'The great
source of pleasure is variety' said Dr Johnson. Medicine offers
great variety and doctors on their part have long contributed
more than medicine to the world around them.

6

Time out but well spent: research and work abroad

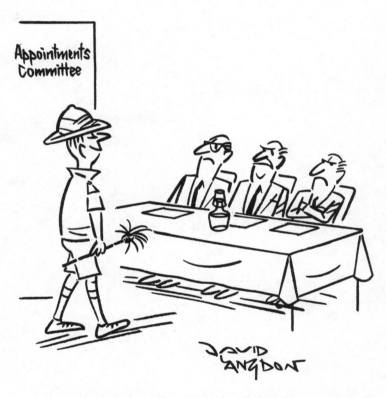

. . . do not on the whole look imaginatively . . .

6

Time out but well spent: research and work abroad

There are several good reasons for temporarily stepping off the direct career ladder. The usual ones are to obtain a rigorous training in laboratory-based research or to work abroad in order to obtain general or special experience with a different perspective. The unusual include taking a year off soon after registration in order to perfect organ playing; the person in mind is now both a consultant physician and one of the handful of doctors who are Fellows of the Royal College of Organists. But the treadmill of specialist training in medicine is becoming demanding to an extent which makes it increasingly difficult to take time out, even for the best of reasons, without losing out. It is still possible and indeed often desirable to take time out but the timing has become critical. The optimum timing may well be different in different specialties and there is not in any case general agreement on what is best. Whatever the professionally and academically most desirable moment, considerations such as the manpower approval as a recognised trainee within a fixed pool may override other considerations.

The general benefits of training in research

Training and experience in research gives a cutting edge to clinical practice and encourages continuing self-education. The importance of an introduction to the acquisition and refinement of new knowledge in medicine has been forcefully expressed by the Committee of Vice Chancellors and Principals of the UK:

> The most important task for medical education is to give students the aptitude and motivation for a lifetime of continuing self education, that will fit them for the practice of medicine well into the next century. They must be taught, and learn, in a context in which they see new knowledge being acquired, assessed and integrated into clinical practice.

For a few, research training at an early stage of their career turns out to be the foundation and inspiration of a lifetime of clinical research in academic posts or in industry.

Intercalated BSc degrees

A first introduction to study in-depth, including the acquisition of the attitudes and methods of clinical research, is conveniently obtained as an undergraduate by means of an intercalated BSc course. This is usually taken at most universities between the pre-clinical and clinical parts of the course, i.e., at the end of the second year. Newcastle has a BMedSci course which can be intercalated then or during the clinical course. London University has introduced an optional intercalated BSc in clinical science during the clinical course, taken at present between the second and final clinical years.

Unfortunately, Local Education Authorities rarely support students for this important and formative year and the Medical Research Council now only supports about 6% of the student intake for this purpose. Universities have found some other sources of support but most medical students taking an intercalated BSc now have to find their own financial support. Students at Oxford and Cambridge are fortunate because their preclinical BA course is three years for all students, the third year offering an educational experience similar to an intercalated BSc.

Research years during 'career' training

Research does not necessarily mean time out but it is very difficult to combine clinical responsibility satisfactorily with the acquisition of a rigorous training in research techniques. A period of fulltime research is an integral part of many specialist training programmes. The outcome is often a thesis for the MD degree. JPAC still has to accept that provided this research period precedes or follows full service training as a 'career' registrar it does not frustrate manpower planning and honorary clinical contracts should therefore not be a problem. No additional doctors are needed to man the service. The entry to specialist training and the output to consultant posts is unaffected. The pool of doctors in training will enlarge to a new steady state and the transit time through the pool will be faster for those spending little or no time in research than for the others. There is no logical reason why 'career' registrar contracts should not be retained on an honorary basis by those who incorporate research within their professional training programme between completion of a 'career' registrar training and entry to the senior registrar grade. Diminishing financial resources are making it increasingly difficult to fund research years off-service but such is the concern that clinical research is going to be seriously harmed by increasingly rigid training programmes that the Medical Research Council and research charities are likely to support the able and determined.

Academic posts give greater in-service research opportunity because academics have a contractual obligation to contribute to their subject through research in addition to teaching and providing a clinical service. NHS training posts neither have a requirement to undertake research nor do they usually provide adequate facilities or time for it in the course of heavy clinical duties. The dilemma of specialist training is how to acquire the necessary clinical skills through practical experience, sufficient knowledge through study to pass essential Royal College or Faculty diplomas and adequate research training and experience to provide the substance for a higher degree.

Research in general practice

For general practice there is no such problem. Neither a higher diploma nor a higher degree is required. On the other hand much is ripe for asking and ready for answering in the setting of general practice and many of the brightest medical graduates enter general practice as their first choice. They might well find that the academic stimulus of research would make their work even more fulfilling, and several prizes are offered nationally for research projects undertaken during vocational training for general practice.

Published research is an essential requirement for career posts in academic units of general practice. A period of research after the completion of a General Practice Vocational Training Scheme (VTS) may in other circumstances hinder rather than help in the acquisition of a principal's post. Prospective practice partners may doubt such an individual's commitment to service, may be sceptical about the value of research to the everyday task of providing a service, or may simply feel threatened by the entry of a bright, questioning young man or woman to the practice. These attitudes are ill-founded and should pass, but their passing will take time. Research fellowships in the field of primary health care are available on a competitive basis from the MRC, Wellcome Trust and other bodies and are normally taken up in academic units. They are best taken soon after the completion of vocational training, before the relatively low salary they offer becomes unacceptable. Training schemes for general practice may be self-constructed provided they are approved and there is no reason why a scheme should not be devised, with help and advice from an academic unit and the Regional Adviser in General Practice, which includes a period of research relevant in its skills to general practice – skills such as epidemiology and medical statistics.

The timing of a period in research

All the clinical medical specialties require the Membership of the Royal Colleges of Physicians of the UK (MRCP(UK)) as an entry qualification and it is best to acquire this diploma before diverting for any reason after qualification, be it research, work abroad or having a baby. Success in the MRCP examination requires both a steady momentum in learning from the time of Finals or preferably even earlier, and as much and as varied clinical experience as possible. The task is harder if posts leave neither time nor energy for private study, are too far removed from the stimulus of a large teaching centre in preparation for the examination, or do not provide broad clinical experience. Single-minded determination to pass the examination at the first possible opportunity is the best policy. The sooner it is passed the better the prospect of a career in a subspecialty of first choice and the greater the time and opportunity to include research as a complementary part of the training.

The most opportune moment for a period in research in most specialties is after obtaining the necessary higher diploma and a good grounding of clinical experience. In other words between the registrar and senior registrar appointments, but there are exceptions (see below). Timing is more difficult in pathology specialties and community medicine because the higher diploma is taken on completion of training. A research project is part of the requirements for the MFCM so that there is a greater incentive to divert during training in community medicine.

For many years, a majority of surgeons intending a career in 'general surgery' as distinct from the specialties, such as orthopaedics, cardiothoracic surgery, urology and neurosurgery, have undertaken a period of research either in a biological laboratory (often part of a surgical department, but not necessarily so) or in the wards, or both. This trend is being taken up in the specialties as competition becomes fiercer and there is a need to offer something extra on one's *curriculum vitae*. The traditional time to undertake this research has been after gaining the fellowship and often also after some post-fellowship experience so that the research fills the gap between the conventional registrar and senior registrar appointment. There are disadvantages in this: once well embarked on professional training it is difficult and unsatisfactory to break away; the registrar now in his or her late twenties or early thirties often has family commitments which interfere with the ability to travel and make it more difficult to live laborious days in the execution of a research project; even if this is achieved, writing up papers and producing a thesis are very difficult after returning to fulltime clinical work; and the new style surgical professional training described above will make a gap for research increasingly difficult to find. In consequence, some surgeons are increasingly tending to take time out for research immediately after the primary fellowship has been achieved. The greater flexibility of the mind in the young has advantages in the increasingly demanding world of biomedical research.

In the current transition period it requires courage, confidence and the appropriate degree both of motivation and support from a supervisor to embark on a year or, increasingly, two years of fulltime research without having any assurance of successful entry into surgical training. There are rare examples, which will probably become more common, of an appointment to a training programme being made but entry deferred until a research project has been completed.

Though courage *is* required to undertake such a course, there is the bonus of having behind one either a significant body of published work or a thesis, or best of all, both. Not only is this ultimately of great personal satisfaction but also, as already mentioned, it may provide the little extra something that will impress those who are seeking to create the next generation of surgeons. In this context it is having achieved a research project and written it up satisfactorily that is the yardstick rather than the field of endeavour that has been pursued. In the current climate of over-supply, must successful applicants for higher surgical training in the most popular branches of surgery will not only have a considerable number of published papers but also will have completed a higher degree, either a PhD or a MD (the MS persists in many universities but has virtually the same meaning as an MD though in some universities – the minority – there is still a clinical/viva). The PhD can be achieved sooner than an MD or MS which traditionally requires at least five years post-registration experience. Though what has been described applies most to the current state of research in relation to general surgery, there is a trend in some of the specialties – orthopaedics in particular – for research and the achievement of a thesis to become essential. It is important at an early stage to find out what is the consensus for the specialty you chose.

Obstetrics and gynaecology, anaesthetics, radiology and psychiatry all have their Royal College diploma examinations at a similar stage of specialty training to surgery, and later than for medicine. With them all the relevant diploma is required in order to gain a senior registrar post. Acquiring the necessary specialist examination knowledge and experience becomes, as with surgery, the first priority for several years, deferring research opportunity until a relatively senior stage in comparison with medical specialties. By this stage, opportunities for research outside academic units are few. Medical Research Council and Wellcome Trust fellowships are the most numerous and also the most highly competitive; various other charitable foundations offer a small number of research fellowships and so does the pharmaceutical industry, although these latter are usually tied to specific projects. Most of these fellowships are advertised in the general medical journals.

In pathology, the long years of prescribed experience leading up to the MRCPath examinations have been a considerable disincentive to research and the usually rapid assumption of consultant responsibility after passing the MRCPath has limited research opportunity. A research thesis will in future be acceptable as part of the requirement for Part 2 of the MRCPath.

There is much to be said for those planning an academic career in medicine for spending two or three years working for a PhD in a basic science department, thereby obtaining a far more rigorous scientific background and training in research techniques than an undergraduate medical education provides. It is highly desirable at the same time to retain some limited clinical responsibility to prevent clinical skills becoming rusty. Current manpower restrictions are making it more difficult to get an honourary clinical contract for this purpose.

The more extensive the clinical experience before embarking on research the less a gap will matter, but even well developed clinical skills need to be practised if they are not to be lost. A limited but outstanding opportunity for combined research and general professional training has recently been introduced by the Medical Research Council in the form of a small number of seven-year training fellowships available in open competition for three years in a basic medical science laboratory and three or four years of clinical training in a personally-tailored programme, not necessarily all undertaken at one institution. Other educational opportunities are being developed both to combine undergraduate medical education with a PhD and to combine postgraduate

specialty training with an MD or PhD in a programme similar to
the MRC seven-year fellowships.

Research publications and presentations

Research should be guided by pertinent questions, should achieve
answers in a reasonable time and should be written up for publication. Publications do not have to be long to be useful, indeed
they should be no longer than necessary to communicate and
demonstrate the essential points. Study the 'Instructions to
Authors' of your chosen journal before writing anything. There is
much to be said for writing the 'Abstract' first to focus the
framework of the paper: what was done and why, what was
found, and what does it mean? The 'Introduction' should be short
– long enough only to set the scene. The 'Methods' section should
describe any new methods so that they can be repeated by others
and should refer by reference only to standard methods used.
'Results' should be tabulated as far as possible and the major ones
highlighted in the text. 'Discussion' should be succinct and not
attempt a complete review of other publications on the topic; it
should arrive at a conclusion as to the significance of the findings.
References quoted should be limited to the strictly necessary and
should not become a showcase for previous personal publications. Write, rewrite, put away for a week or two then reread and
if necessary rewrite. Keep the language as simple and as clear as
possible. Ask your friends to read and criticise. Be prepared to
have your work torn to pieces; bury your pride and enjoy the
excitement of learning and doing better all the time.

It is also important to show your face, to present and defend
your research work at scientific meetings, initially at departmental seminars but later further afield at general societies such as
the Medical Research Society, the Surgical Research Society or a
specialist society. International meetings are on the whole less
cost effective in critically refining ideas, unless arranged as small
seminars limited to experts in the field, but they lead to a wider
and often more stimulating world.

The traditional advice to speakers still applies, whether in
research or in case presentations. Stand up, speak up and sit
down. Prepare legible slides without too much on them. Write

large on overhead transparencies; spell correctly. If using an overhead projector and it cannot be adjusted to project over your head, stand back so that the screen can be seen and you can point to it. Be quite clear of the nature of the audience and therefore of the level at which your presentation should be pitched.

Service and study abroad

Many doctors have a yearning to spend time abroad. While undoubtedly educating in the broadest sense, few posts in developing countries offer approved postgraduate training for Royal College and Faculty diplomas because of the relative lack of supervision and shortage of facilities. On the other hand they provide an opportunity to contribute much needed medical skill and a perspective on the limitations of Western medicine in a global context. But if aiming for any specialty other than general practice, a period in the Third World interrupts diplomas. If a year is taken abroad after obtaining a higher diploma it needs to have a specific purpose if it is not to hinder rather than help in the acquisition of a senior registrar post, except perhaps in accident and emergency, and in infectious diseases. Appointments committees do not on the whole look imaginatively on missionary spirit or humanitarian concern.

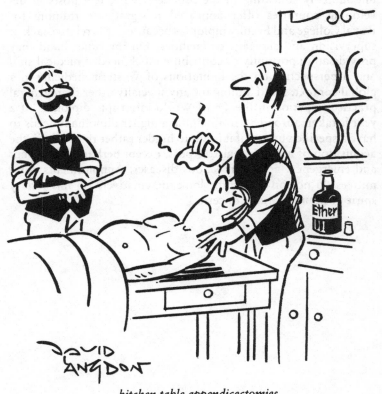

... kitchen table appendicectomies ...

7

Clinical practice outside hospital

General practice

My father's worn brass plate, stolen alas the day he retired, read 'W. Richards, MB BChir MRCS, LRCP, Physician and Surgeon', pretentious by today's standards but a good description of the whole doctor his generation was. He did not think to mention that he was an obstetrician too, for that was just part of the domiciliary job. Surgery was the smaller role and steadily diminished: kitchen table appendicectomies, with a partner giving the ether anaesthetic, did not outlast the World War II, but minor surgery continued. Medicine was the core of the job.

His father's draper's shop in a Devonshire country town had emblazoned across the whitewashed front 'Richards for Sterling Service', not a bad motto for a future general practitioner, discretely omitting the last part of the slogan which said 'Ready Money'. That in fact was how much of his general practice was conducted, at least amongst his poorer patients, who paid little but usually something.

Getting to Cambridge from Grammar School, staying the course and collecting together sufficient funds to buy a practice in a London suburb cost him much application and his inheritance in advance. General practice was his life, an unambitious, dogged, selfless life; there were many like him. He was practically always available: Thursday was his half-day and by four, five or six o'clock he would usually have extricated himself from the practice to take my mother out for the evening. Sunday afternoon and evening were generally free unless he was worried about any patients and, in any case, there was always 'booking' to catch up with. There were surgeries morning and evening for an hour or two every day except Thursday evening and Sunday, usually overrunning, and 15–20 home visits every day and a few on Sunday. He was often called out at night.

Those arrogant enough to think that holism is something new should have seen the little sign hanging on the wall behind his black oak pigeon-holed desk: 'Don't Worry It May Not Happen'. He knew that most illness required no medicine and that he had nothing effective for most of the conditions which did. He knew what worked and what did not and had a good idea why. He could not abide quackery, of which there was (and still is) plenty about.

His therapeutic career had got off to a shaky start in Finals at Cambridge: when asked the dose of senna his reply received the riposte 'That, my boy, would not move the bowels of a common house fly'. His little white boxes of red, blue, green, brown and white-coated aspirins were used with great discrimination: red usually worked best. He also had an impish hunch that unpleasant mixtures were the most effective. In 1938 he received a letter from a patient describing a hunt through his house for a 'terrible odour' which even the builders who were called in emergency could not localise until 'somebody shouted – "my goodness, what's in this glass" – and my little wife disclosed it was the medicine ... I'm better now Doctor, must I have more medicine?'

A keen sense of urgency in clinical diagnosis was always with him and he had an excellent nose for a surgical case; he also knew which surgeon to turn to for rapid help. The partnership between specialist and general practitioner was both personal and effective in those days. He did not call for help unnecessarily and he did not panic. Told one day urgently by an anxious mother that Johnny had swallowed a silver threepenny piece he replied calmly that it was a pity Lloyd George was dead. Pressed for an explanation he replied 'He could get money out of anyone'. His prescription was porridge.

Acute medical crises were common too. Sulphonamides transformed his practice and lengthened the lives of many of his patients; penicillin, a few years later, was magical. But the introduction of these effective treatments neither made him careless in diagnosis nor profligate in treatment. He was a first-rate doctor and an excellent diagnostician.

He had no secretarial support and kept his own accounts, using an accountant only for the auditing. Patients were charged what he estimated they could afford – around 1950 that was between sixpence (2 ½p) and five shillings (25p) for a home visit; some paid nothing. He was worried that the introduction of a free NHS might destroy the relationship between doctor and patient and that doctors would be taken for granted. His rough and ready financial socialism (not to be confused with his politics, for he was an old-fashioned Liberal) beggared no one, except perhaps himself, and he could always arrange a home visit from a specialist for very little if necessary, or a consultation at hospital for nothing.

The cost of his lifetime of devotion to his patients fell on himself (but it was his life and he would not have changed it) and on his wife, my mother, who was slave to telephone and surgeries. She lived for Thursday evenings and the month's holiday in August, except that being married to a homing West Country pigeon, holidays were somewhat lacking in diversity.

General practice has changed almost out of recognition in its terms and its trappings in a short time, but the reason for mentioning how it used to be is to emphasise that the philosophy of the best practice remains the same. To be readily available is the first requirement; the second is to listen, to examine, and to think in the context of the patient's environment, taking urgent action if necessary; the third is to provide continuity of care.

Good practice organisation has relieved much of the domestic burden. Many of the nursing tasks have been taken over by practice nurses and the administration by a practice manager. A knowledge of the business side of running a practice and of how the remuneration is built up from a mixture of capitation fees, practice allowances and item-of-service payments must be acquired in due course but can properly wait until vocational training.

Partnerships

When considering entering a partnership advice must be taken to avoid pitfalls, and not from future partners because they, subconsciously no doubt, have their own nests to line, but from the BMA, a medical defence society or a lawyer skilled in partnership agreements. You really cannot be too careful: I recall a much respected senior partner who calmly told his junior partner that his parity of earnings in the practice would have to be delayed because he, the senior partner, had more expensive school fees to pay. The matters which need formal definition and agreement include those listed in Table 7.1

Table 7.1. Matters requiring formal definition in partnership agreement[23]

1. Initial assets of the partnership.
2. Respective shares of profits and losses.
3. A breakdown of which expenses and earnings belong to the practice and which to the individual partner.
4. Formal arrangements about holiday, study leave and number of partners allowed to be away at one time.
5. Time devoted by partners to outside appointments.
6. Maternity/paternity leave provision.
7. Arrangements for sickness insurance to cover the cost of locums etc.
8. Arrangements for the partnership if one partner leaves, dies or becomes bankrupt.

The nature of the task

General practice is family medicine, a setting which itself provides the clues to so much ill health. For this reason in particular, general practice is more satisfying and effective in a stable, settled community than in an area in which people are rootless, restless and on their own, without the support of family and friends. Provision of primary care to the washed up and washed out is an important but rather different challenge although still probably better undertaken by general practitioners than by hospitals.

The task of general practitioners is to hold the front line, partly in promoting health and partly by coping with illness of all sorts, providing sympathy, encouragement, explanation and, when necessary, treatment. More serious illness has to be recognised for what it is and the patient passed on (like Oscar Wilde's 'good advice') for further opinion or investigation. Immunisations and family planning are an important part of health promotion and health education. Encouragement of the avoidance of smoking and of heavy drinking are another aspect and demand a certain standard of example by the doctor. The key feature of British medicine is a personal doctor, the general practitioner, able to cross the boundaries between narrow specialisms, a concept hotly attacked when introduced in the 1820s but defended in these words in 1830:

> the general practitioner ... does not, when called upon, stop to inquire if his patient is affected with a medical or a surgical disorder; he feels himself doubly armed, for either emergency ... we do not want to borrow a consequence from the mere name of surgeon or doctor, we hope to be able to assert our consequence by our utility ... the title of general practitioner does not, I humbly assert, degrade us. A man may degrade a title, but the title cannot degrade the man.[24]

Home visits have become a smaller part of a general practitioner's work; surgeries have increased in proportion. Continuity of care is one of the most important features of good medical practice. No doctor can reasonably or safely be on duty all the time. Most now work in group practices, where supporting staff come to know all the frequent attenders whichever doctor they see and where the partnership gets to know, discuss and cover each other's patients. With a team approach to continuity of care within the reach of most doctors, the use of anonymous deputising services seems very second best, but in inner-city communities where up to 40% of a doctor's patients change every year and visiting at night is hazardous, the situation is complicated. It is not, however, only a general practitioner's knowledge and skill but his or her dedication and total identification with patients' welfare which has been at the heart of the special relationship between general practitioner, individual patients and the community. It is difficult to see how without continuity of care this special relationship can survive.

Within a group practice, partners often develop different special expertise and to some extent refer patients to each other. This degree of specialisation, together possibly with sessions as a clinical assistant in hospital, offers an agreeable balance between generalism and specialism. The medical and supporting staff of a group practice form a multidisciplinary team, providing a round-the-clock service which they all believe to be worthwhile and which for all in their different ways is a satisfying way of life.

General practice is not, however, a bed of roses. The work is as much pastoral as medical and much is routine, although much of the routine is never quite the same. Some rural practices still provide a dispensing service, which provides additional interest and income; dispensing has long since ceased to be an apothecary's art. A few patients are unreasonably demanding and even hostile; the general practitioner's only remedy *in extremis* is to ask the Family Practitioner Committee (FPC) to remove a patient from his list. Night work is not generally very heavy but may become a burden, especially in violent inner-city areas and as the doctor ages.

Attractions of general practice include being part of the local community, working close to home, seeing the patient in the context of the family circle, the satisfaction of seeing patients gratefully recover from common ailments as well as from the occasional more serious illness, and being as much a family friend as medical adviser. Above all, general practice offers the opportunity to settle into a permanent home in a chosen area at an earlier stage than with a hospital career. Even after practice expenses (many of which are substantially reimbursed by the FPC), earnings are generally higher and reach a sufficient level in time to meet the peak period of family demands. Domestic commitments are more readily fitted in and around general practice, fulltime or part-time. Some doctors do not however, readily come to terms with the wide remit of general practice and are better suited to narrower specialisation in hospital.

Pathways of training

Two training pathways lead to a principal's post in general practice. Most doctors entering general practice undertake an accident and emergency post before starting the formal training programme. One alternative is a formal three-year Vocational Training Scheme (VTS). Two years are spent in SHO posts in hospital disciplines particularly relevant to general practice. One year is spent as a trainee in a practice under the supervision of General Practice Trainer, a general practitioner who has been recognised by the Joint Committee on Postgraduate Training in Royal College of General Practitioners on account of his interest, the high standard of his practice, a short period of formal training and attendance at continuing short courses. The trainer usually holds regular seminars with the trainee to discuss issues in general practice and specific patients. While working in practice the trainee's salary is higher than in hospital and a car allowance is payable. The work is essentially that of an assistant taking a share of all aspects of the work, including home visits and night calls but with the trainer always readily available for advice and support. The other pathway is through a similar but self-arranged series of posts which offer a similar pattern of training. Popular specialties in the programmes include obstetrics, paediatrics and psychiatry.

Half-day release schemes centred on the local postgraduate medical centre are a feature of Vocational Training Schemes for general practice. Seminars cover a wide range of topics such as practice management, clinical problems, therapeutics, patients' views, ethnic minorities and their customs, complementary therapies, health promotion and relating to problem patients. These meetings are also an excellent opportunity for trainees to discuss their experiences together with each other and with their trainers.

Certificates of prescribed or equivalent service

About 40% of doctors are aiming for a career in general practice by the time they complete their preregistration posts and about half of all medical graduates eventually become GPs. The only essential qualification in addition to a medical degree is either a Certificate of Prescribed Experience on completion of an approved VTS or a Certificate of Equivalent Experience on the basis of a similar but self-arranged programme accepted by the Joint Committee on Higher Medical Training in General Practice as equivalent to a VTS. Part-time training is recognised both for the hospital and the GP components of the training programme, provided it amounts to at least five sessions per week. Posts in a VTS may be shared. Supernumerary part-time posts may be arranged and funded by a Regional Health Authority. All GP training posts must be approved by the Royal College of General Practitioners. If contemplating part-time training, discuss personal plans with either the Regional Adviser in General Practice or with the Regional Postgraduate Dean, whose address is obtainable from any hospital Clinical Tutor or from a medical school's Postgraduate Subdean.

A higher diploma is not essential for general practice but many entrants obtain the DCH (Diploma of Child Health), DCCH (Diploma in Community and Child Health) or the MRCP. For a general practitioner who wishes to be on the Obstetric List the DRCOG (Diploma of the Royal College of Obstetricians and Gynaecologists) is essential. Membership of the Royal College of General Practitioners is also a sensible investment and may become mandatory in due course.

Finding a practice

Towards the end of the VTS, feelers must be put out for a permanent position in a practice. Often vacancies coming up locally are made known to the trainers and it is sensible to enter a VTS in an area in which you would wish to settle. Sometimes it may be necessary to look further afield by responding to advertisements in the journals or by following up word-of-mouth information. It is now usual to go straight for a principal's post rather than to become a salaried assistant in one practice before looking for a partnership in another. It is usual for the first year to be probationary and for the remuneration to be less than an equal share of the practice profits. Once the appointment is confirmed as mutually satisfactory the new partner should proceed rapidly to parity of income. Some doctors, especially married women with heavy domestic commitments, may prefer to take sessional work in a practice, usually only clinic work without visits or night calls, in which case they work on a salaried sessional basis.

The new partner is likely to be considered fair game by the chronically dissatisfied patients of the practice who welcome the opportunity to pour out their woes to a doctor they have not yet exhausted. As his or her list is initially likely to be smaller than that of the long-established partners most of the acute new patients may come to the new partner. While these activities are developing in the surgery a number of questions need to be resolved at home concerning the relationship between the doctor's spouse and the practice responsibilities, not least whether calls will be taken by the one at home or by answerphone and bleep. As with the practice agreement, arrangements at home need to be clearly sorted out to prevent tensions and trouble later.

The challenge and opportunity of contributing by research to the future of general practice, or of taking part in local government as a councillor, or of becoming a magistrate are such that the danger of a mid-life crisis in the relative professional isolation of general practice can readily be overcome by diversification of contribution both to the community and to the discipline.

Community health

Community health does not currently belong in a list of specialist careers in medicine, and is mentioned only to avoid confusion. Clinical Medical Officers (CMO) and Senior Clinical Medical Officers (SCMO) undertake sessional work in a community setting in a disparate collection of clinics, each important in its own way, but not providing a permanent career appointment. They offer convenient, useful and, generally, part-time employment, and are posts which for the latter reason in particular are predominantly held by women doctors. The posts are under review and may either be subsumed into general practice or may possibly be refashioned as part of a new area of consultant responsibility with an appropriate postgraduate training programme. For many of the areas covered, previous appropriate experience and diploma qualification (such as the DCCH) would clearly be most appropriate. The areas covered are shown in Table 7.2.

Table 7.2. Areas of sessional work in community health

Child health including school health service
Family planning
Audiology
Geriatrics
Mental health
Antenatal and postnatal clinics
Well-woman clinics

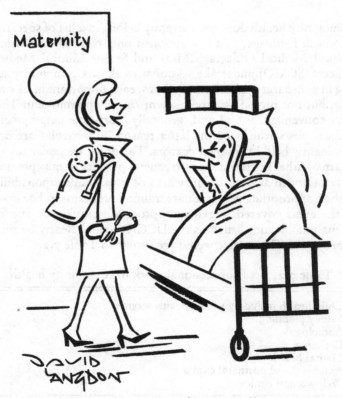

'And how are we this morning?'

8

Clinical practice in hospital: higher training programmes and work patterns

Medical specialties (Table 8.1)

The specialties included officially in this term and the number of consultants in each on 30th September, 1987, are shown in Table 8.1. Numbers are gradually increasing in all specialties but not yet at the promised rate of 2% per annum. The initial pathway for all specialties except paediatrics is the same, namely a series of SHO posts in general medicine and some of its specialties as part of general professional training. Sometimes these posts are linked in a rotation of three or four posts on a balanced and geographically compact scheme; at other times it is necessary to find a series of separate posts when and where one can. Most medical registrar posts combine general medicine with a variable component of specialisation.

General medicine

General medicine covers the whole range of medical conditions at their relatively undifferentiated or undiagnosed stage, especially in their emergency presentations, besides the care of patients with multisystem diseases. It forms the core of consultant physician work at District General Hospitals for the staff is too small to contain specialists in every specialty and most inpatients are admitted as an acute emergency. Even outpatient referrals from general practitioners need a widely based consultant opinion in order to narrow the diagnosis to a particular system, before referral or when necessary to a more specialised colleague.

With the exception of specialties such as dermatology, cardiology and rheumatology (which tend to have purely specialist posts at registrar level) specialisation in medicine starts in earnest at the senior registrar stage. Doctors are now specialising earlier with the result that general professional training may soon be largely confined to SHO posts. But a strand of general responsibility usually continues throughout training: even at senior registrar level, subspecialty experience in, for example, cardiology, endocrinology, gastroenterology, nephrology, clinical pharmacology, infectious diseases or thoracic medicine, is usually combined with acute general medical intaking experience – an entirely appropriate training for the clinical demands upon most District General Hospital consultant physicians. Formal specialist accreditation is consequently often earned in both the subspecialty and in general medicine after three or four years as a senior registrar.

Work patterns in medical training

The general responsibilities of SHOs, registrars and senior registrars are similar but the most junior staff undertake more of the day-to-day practical continuity, while the senior registrar has a larger advisory role and carries more responsibility. Emergency admitting duty is likely to be on a rota of between 1 in 3 and 1 in 5, sometimes with registrar and senior registrar (if there are both) alternating in their resident backup duty to the house physician and SHO (if there is one). Senior registrars usually have prime responsibility for arranging duty rotas and they provide cover for consultants on leave, usually in addition to their normal responsibilities. Where there is no senior registrar the registrar is likely to assume these roles with appropriate cover from the remaining consultants.

There is much else for the senior registrar to do. There will be a business round with the other junior staff five days a week with a watching brief for any particularly sick patients over the weekend, even when not formally on duty. Twice a week routinely, and more frequently on intake, there will be a round with

Table 8.1. Medical specialties in England and Wales, 1987[2]

	Consultants	
	Total	% Female
General medicine	1295	4.6
Cardiology	136	5.9
Diabetes and endocrinology	30	6.7
Gastroenterology	34	2.9
Nephrology	67	4.5
Thoracic medicine	105	8.6
Geriatric medicine	487	11.9
Audiology	15	33.3
Clinical genetics	37	29.7
Clinical neurophysiology	52	21.2
Clinical pharmacology and therapeutics	42	4.8
Clinical physiology	23	0
Dermatology	237	21.1
Genito-urinary medicine	134	16.4
Oncology	34	8.8
Infectious diseases	31	0
Neurology	179	3.4
Rheumatology	234	12.0
Paediatrics	660	22.4
Paediatric neurology	15	20.0

the consultant. Undergraduate teaching on selected patients once or twice a week is a good way of learning oneself besides the stimulus of any lecture or seminar teaching. Usually a clinical meeting for all the medical firms is held weekly ('staff round'). The quality of the 'staff round' and of the presentations by the more junior members of the firm is a good indicator of the commitment, influence and ability of the senior registrar. At least two out-patient clinics are likely weekly, one general and one subspecialty. Then there should be a deaths and discharges meeting for the whole firm weekly, postmortem examinations to attend, inpatient summaries to dictate and occasional administrative committee meetings to attend. Besides these duties the senior registrar is expected to have a day each week for private study and research leading to publications and, if not completed already, to an MD thesis.

Medical subspecialties

Practically all consultant physicians, most of whom would describe themselves as general physicians, have an area of special interest and expertise. Others are specialists in a narrow field in which they spend all their time.

Cardiologists spend much of their time in investigation by cardiac catheterisation and, increasingly, treating coronary artery stenosis by angioplasty. They report on cardiac ultrasonography, isotope scans, exercise tests and resting cardiographs. Inpatient work is dominated by ischaemic heart disease; outpatient work by the diagnosis of chest pains and the continuing care in partnership with general practitioners of a decreasing number of patients with old rheumatic valvular disease, patients in and out of heart failure and follow up of those who have had cardiac surgery.

Endocrinologists spend much of their time planning, arranging and undertaking day investigation of suspected endocrine disease. Gastroenterologists have a heavy diagnostic load of upper and lower gastrointestinal fibre-optic endoscopies, small bowel biopsies and liver biopsies to perform. Their inpatient work covers a wide variety of upper and lower bowel disease, particularly peptic ulceration, inflammatory bowel disease and cancer. Gastroenterology is a specialty which calls for close partnership between physician and surgeon and it is becoming common practice to have joint units. Outpatient clinics are dominated by patients with abdominal pains and disordered bowel habit. Chronic liver disease also finds its way to the gastroenterologists, except in large, highly specialised hospitals which have a specialist hepatologist.

Thoracic medicine, like other subspecialties such as cardiology and gastroenterology, covers intensively one end of a spectrum of disease much of which is considered everyday acute general medicine: the more difficult diagnostic or therapeutic respiratory problems come the way of the specialised chest physician. After years of being an exclusive respiratory and largely clinic-based specialty, younger specialists in thoracic medicine seem on the whole to prefer to combine their subspecialty with continuing involvement in general medicine. The old-style chest clinic physician, conducting annual reviews of patients who had tuberculosis long ago or of patients with severe chronic but stable respiratory disease, are largely a memory of the past, although most acute tuberculosis still comes to the chest physicians and they also are responsible for case contact follow up.

Nephrology has become increasingly identified with the management of chronic renal failure by intermittent haemodialysis, continuous ambulatory peritoneal dialysis or renal transplantation. The management of acute renal failure is a less common but important role and is where the subspecialty really started. The investigation and treatment of hypertension more often falls to the nephrologist than the cardiologist but clinical pharmacologists have made determined bids for hypertension and have made substantial contributions. Determination of the significance of proteinuria and the investigation of impaired renal function are the bread and butter of new consultations in renal clinics. Surgically remediable obstructive renal disease, renal calculi and disorders of bladder function provide important areas of joint medical and surgical collaboration and joint units between nephrologists and urologists make much sense.

Infectious diseases is the subspecialty polymath of medicine, providing for all ages, involving all body systems and covering all hours. Great diagnostic skill is involved in making the necessary rapid diagnoses and especially in recognising the need for urgent investigation and treatment, including emergency surgery on rare occasions. Knowledge and experience must range from the mundane to the exotic, from the temperate to the tropical. The proper management of infectious diseases calls for urgent and often difficult decisions. Opportunities for training in the specialty are few in the UK but more numerous in the USA. The emergence of HIV has suddenly made infectious diseases a growth specialty. Genitourinary medicine (sexually transmitted diseases) in particular has expanded. Clinical immunology has also expanded but it remains a very small specialty and the opportunities for training are even smaller than in infectious diseases (see p. 132).

Neurology has been revolutionised and to a substantial extent diagnostically demystified by the introduction of computerised tomography (CT) scans and magnetic resonance imaging (MRI). Many areas remain, however, in which the traditional diagnostic skills and judgements are important and neurologists spend much time giving peripatetic opinions. Most neurologists have to cover a wide geographical area but practically all of them have a base in a combined neurological and neurosurgical centre from which they fan out like the spokes of a wheel. Outpatient work tends to be dominated by headaches and epilepsy; inpatient work by cerebral tumours and cerebrovascular disease.

Backache and nonspecific joint pains are the staple diet of rheumatologists, for whom classical, deforming rheumatoid arthritis remains an important but relatively minor part of their work. Rehabilitation of patients with all sorts of disabilities has become a particular interest of some doctors in this field, sometimes identified as specialists in rheumatology and rehabilitation in multidisciplinary rehabilitation units. The two interests seem to be going their separate ways and a training in the much-needed cinderella sub-specialty of rehabilitation is hard to come by.

Dermatology, like neurology, is thinly spread across the country; it is even more strongly outpatient based and dermatologists generally work at several hospitals. It is a specialty in the process of finding its scientific feet, although many dermatological diagnoses remain purely descriptive and their treatment empirical. A few common and literally irritating conditions account for a substantial part of the day to day work. Many systemic diseases present with skin manifestations, adding further diagnostic interest to the dermatologist's work. Diagnostic techniques, such as skin biopsy are relatively straightforward and the hours are convenient. On the other hand skin diseases cause much discomfort, misery and frustration and some misery may even cause skin disease. The dermatologist therefore needs to be a good doctor in the widest sense if patients, especially the chronic ones, are to be substantially helped.

Medical oncology, the chemotherapeutic arm of radiotherapy (see p. 138), which is sometimes separate and sometimes a part of radiotherapy, is an emotionally demanding field suitable for determined optimists. The diagnostic skills required are as much for the detection and management of complications of treatment as for the cancer itself. The underlying disease has usually been diagnosed before the patient is referred to an oncologist but the hazards of cancer chemotherapy are great. Rapid diagnosis of treatable complications of cancer or its treatment together with support and encouragement of patients and their families in a heartbreaking situation are, however, very worthwhile. Cures are rare but they do happen. Some senior registrars in this field and in radiotherapy become consultants working full time in the 'continuing care' of patients with advanced cancer, based in hospital but currently a small subspecialty.

Other subspecialties listed in Table 8.1 such as clinical genetics, clinical neurophysiology and clinical physiology are small specialties which require a solid scientific background and laboratory training; they are confined to a few large centres. Clinical genetics is a growth area but it starts from a very small base.

Paediatrics (child health) is in many ways a different art to adult medicine. It contains many of the subspecialty interests developed in adult medicine but they are much smaller disciplines within paediatrics. The key differences between medicine for adults and for children include the much greater dependence in paediatrics on other family members, especially parents, for details of the history; special patience and skill needed to calm, reassure and win the confidence of children; the technically, emotionally and physically demanding care of neonates; and the wide but thin spread of paediatric services across the country in relation to the relatively small number of both senior and junior staff, which imposes a substantial burden of emergency cover on consultants (especially for neonatal work), often at more than one hospital. Paediatrics is one of the most demanding of medical subspecialties: it says much for its interest and the commitment of those who would enter it that it is one of the most oversubscribed.

Geriatrics, the care of the elderly, is essentially general medicine for the elderly, for which the common core of general professional training for medical subspecialties is entirely suitable. Geriatric posts begin at registrar or even at senior registrar level, but emphasise the prevention of disability and the rehabilitation and independence of the elderly. Successful practice of the specialty requires a multidisciplinary team working both in hospital and in patients' homes to provide the support which they need; the skills required are both managerial and medical.

For both the general physicians and geriatricians to provide separate emergency intake services at night is expensive and wasteful of scarce resources. Increasingly the tendency is either for the physicians for the elderly to participate in the general medical night rota or to leave the night work to the general physicians. Elderly patients form a large proportion of the work of most doctors and general physicians are no exception. The age cutoff above which patients are usually admitted directly under the care of geriatricians varies and is usually about 80, although many of their patients are younger. Domiciliary visits at the request of general practitioners form a large part of the work.

A period of training in and through clinical research including training in laboratory methods is an important part of postgraduate education in all medical specialties, as indeed in most other disciplines. Only by asking and attempting to answer questions does an appropriately humble and critical view of the current state of understanding of disease and its treatment develop. The timing and nature of this component of postgraduate medical education has already been considered (see Chapter 6).

Academic medicine

In all the medical subspecialties an academic career is possible although in the smallest specialties the number of posts is vanishingly small. On the whole, university posts offer an intellectually more stimulating environment and a wider world. Clinical academics have a smaller (but still considerable) service load which allows more time for research and teaching. Career earnings are in general smaller than in the NHS (although the basic salary is linked) and substantially smaller than colleagues with a private practice. The number of university posts has probably fallen

Table 8.2. Surgical specialties in England and Wales, 1987[2]

	Consultants	
	Total	% Female
General surgery	954	0.6
Cardiothoracic surgery	120	2.5
Otolaryngology	381	3.1
Neurosurgery	98	1.0
Ophthalmology	442	8.1
Paediatric surgery	37	8.1
Plastic surgery	100	4.0
Trauma and orthopaedic	711	0.6
Urology	201	2.0

about as low as it can if academic medicine is to remain viable. On that basis and considering the relative financial disadvantage of an academic career, prospects for appointment of appropriately interested doctors to academic posts are only likely to improve in the medium to long term. Neither NHS posts nor new appointments to academic posts give absolute security but both are about as secure as any job can be in economically and politically uncertain times.

Surgical specialties (Table 8.2)

Surgery is a long, hard, competitive road, often with heavy emergency duties and few opportunities for part-time involvement. It is particularly difficult to combine surgical training with substantial home commitments and women are poorly represented at consultant level in general surgery or the 'major' disciplines such as orthopaedics, cardiothoracic surgery and urology.

Work patterns in surgical training

Registrar posts are nearly always busy and this clinical involvement is usually combined with the need to achieve a professional qualification. There is relatively little time or opportunity during such appointments to undertake formal research but there are chances of doing some clinically-based projects or for writing up case reports for publication. Such opportunities should be seized because selection committees for higher surgical training will expect a publication record. If possible, papers should have a bearing on the trainee's ultimate specialty choice.

The work of a senior registrar has been described as 'consultant work at nonconsultant hours for nonconsultant pay'. In fact, with a large number of extra duty payments, senior registrars may earn as much, or even more, than junior consultants to an extent that the former are sometimes reluctant to become consultants or at least become very choosey about the posts for which they apply. All senior registrar posts in surgery are based on teaching hospitals and there is nearly always a rotation committee which programmes the trainees through a cluster of hospitals to ensure a mix of Teaching and District General Hospitals and of special clinical exposure. It is important in applying for a post to ensure that it offers the components of training that are desired. Some programmes have special arrangements for several months or even a year's travel or special assignment so that more advanced skills can be obtained or an area of research relevant to the chosen specialty pursued. To get on such a training programme is obviously ideal.

Besides having virtual consultant responsibility in the operating theatre and the clinic, a senior registrar has a managerial role in the unit to which he is attached and is a member of various District committees. Special management training courses are gradually being introduced and should be actively sought out.

Finally, after three to four years in the grade (the amount depends on how much retrospective recognition is given for post-fellowship registrar experience and for research – usually no more than a year), accreditation is awarded by the Joint Committee on Higher Surgical Training acting on the advice of its various specialty subcommittees. In theory it is not possible to become a consultant until such accreditation is achieved but it is not unusual to begin to apply when accreditation is 'in the offing' as competition is so severe in many subspecialties of surgery.

General surgery

General surgery is still the largest branch of surgery (see Table 8.2) and, in addition to giving the basic training for a large number of those who will ultimately specialise in another field, is becoming both specialised and diversified in its own right as technical demands increase. Special interests of general surgeons may be organ- or system-based such as the stomach and duodenum, the large bowel, the pancreas, the hepatobiliary tree, the vascular or the endocrine systems. Alternatively they may be disease-based as with surgical oncology. It can be expected that some of the above mentioned subspecialties will become independent over the next two decades.

Surgical subspecialties

Otolaryngology, ophthalmology and to a lesser extent plastic surgery lend themselves better to a training and consultant practice with predictable hours and good prospects for part-time or shared posts but even ophthalmology which has the highest percentage of women consultants of the three contains fewer than 10% of women. One reason is that consultant figures reflect entry to the profession 15 or more years ago at which time only 20% of the undergraduates were women.

Ophthalmology provides a nice balance of surgery and medicine, some of the work being operative but much of it concerning the physics of disordered vision and medical conditions affecting the eye, internally, externally or both. Diabetes is responsible for one substantial area of work of an essentially nonsurgical nature, intervention when necessary usually being by laser treatment. Ophthalmology is very much outpatient-based.

Otolaryngology (ENT) likewise is a special world of its own. It is strongly outpatient-based and straddles surgery and medicine. The surgical aspects range from major head and neck surgery (as a result of cancer or accidental injury) usually carried out in conjunction with plastic surgeons, through tonsillectomy to microsurgery of the middle ear. Antibiotics have largely banished mastoidectomy and greatly reduced the incidence of tonsillectomy, although the operation still has a legitimate place. A substantial part of the medically- and physiologically-based work of ENT surgeons concerns allergic disease of the sinuses and upper airways and the assessment and remedy of hearing disorders. There is currently much interest in new implantable hearing aids and this aspect should grow. Emergency work commonly includes staunching epistaxis and, less frequently but critically, tracheostomy, a procedure which every general surgeon must be able to perform (and even physicians in dire emergency) but which ENT surgeons do better.

Cardiothoracic surgery is in some places one specialty and in others two, with surgeons concentrating either on the heart or on diseases of the lungs and the oesophagus. Thoracic surgeons – that is those in the second group – were nearly put out of business by the demise of tuberculosis but carcinoma of the bronchus for a time filled the gap. Now, although preventive medicine has yet to make a substantial impact, cancer chemotherapy and new insights into the relative merits of radiotherapy and surgery for bronchial carcinoma have reduced the indications for surgery. Oesophageal surgery is usually undertaken by chest surgeons but some general surgeons, especially surgical oncologists and upper gastrointestinal tract surgeons, regard the oesophagus as within their territory. With the decline in rheumatic heart disease, cardiac surgery has become dominated by coronary artery bypass procedures.

Orthopaedic and traumatic surgery

Until recently most Accident and Emergency Departments were run by orthopaedic surgeons because of the large number of skeletal injuries that passed through them. However there is now a separate discipline of emergency medicine which recruits directors for A & E Departments from surgery, medicine and anaesthesia (see p. 118), though orthopaedic surgeons deal with much of the outpatient and all the impatient trauma relevant to their specialty. Orthopaedics is now almost as large a specialty as general surgery and continues to grow because of an aging population subject to accidents and degenerative diseases. At the time of writing orthopaedics and ENT surgery are the only two expanding surgical subspecialties in the UK. Orthopaedics shares a similar pattern of initial experience and higher qualifications with general surgery, although more time may be spent during basic training in specifically orthopaedic posts. Part of the work is driven by a never-ending stream of trauma, largely derived both from road traffic and domestic accidents and which generates a heavy emergency load. Of the remainder, in addition to traditional corrective skeletal and tendon surgery, there have been sophisticated technical advances in fields such as brachial plexus surgery and joint replacement, the latter spurred on by cooperation with bioengineers.

Urologists usually work in close collaboration with nephrologists. Although much of their work is concerned with prostatic obstruction and bladder cancer, a very wide range of disease comes their way including conditions which require reconstructive operations on the urinary tract. The introduction of dynamic studies of bladder function has added dysfunction. Lithotripsy has, on the other hand, simplified much of the surgery of renal calculi. Traditionally urologists have also been associated with renal transplantation for end-stage renal failure and for some of the technical aspects of dialysis for this condition. However, with the extension of transplantation into the heart and liver, there is gradually emerging a subspecialty of transplantation surgery and this process may well accelerate.

Neurosurgery is a relatively small but very demanding sub-specialty with a substantial emergency load of trauma and many other urgent cranial and spinal operations. The training ideally includes a period in neurology. Further, the medical care of post-operative neurosurgical patients is often as critical to survival as the operation itself, and much of this is in the hands of the neurosurgeons themselves. Neurosurgery is almost completely confined to special regional centres. Paediatric surgery is subdiv-ided into similar subspecialties as adult surgery. In its own right it is a much smaller specialty than the other major branches and is largely confined to children's hospitals. Many children are either operated upon by the adult specialist for their condition or by general surgeons.

Plastic surgery is also a small subspecialty – though there are some prospects of future growth – usually entailing a peripatetic sessional way of life. Burns are the major source of the recon-structive work but major cancer surgery and trauma are others. Cosmetic surgery (now regarded as ethically part of the plastic surgeon's work) is an artistic, creative area of work but under-taken for patients who are often very difficult if not impossible to please; it can be very remunerative.

Academic surgery: the clinical practice of those who are employed by universities is integrated into the NHS and in conse-quence the training programmes are very broadly the same whether the individual intends a consultant appointment in the NHS or to become a Senior Lecturer and thence proceed to a Readership or Professorship. Most academic posts in surgery are in general surgery. Of all aspects of surgical advancement this is the most competitive and requires additional research and publication over and above that already necessary for ordinary advancement. Private practice opportunities for university employees are usually more restricted by either regulations (see p. 165) or the demands of teaching, administration and research but there is the possibility of remunerative consultative duties and the financial rewards of writing can also on occasion be considerable.

Table 8.3 Accident and Emergency in England and Wales, 1987[2]

	Consultants	
	Total	% Female
Accident and emergency	190	8.9

Accident and emergency (Table 8.3)

Accident and Emergency (A & E) departments are the shop window of hospitals and the front line trenches of the acute services they provide. For many years their direction was looked upon as a part-time responsibility of specialists in other disciplines, usually an orthopaedic surgeon, whose major interest and commitments lay elsewhere. A & E is at last becoming appropriately recognised as a separate and specific discipline, not by virtue of any particular techniques employed or diseases addressed but because of the situation, mix and unpredictability of the task and the very wide range of skills needed to accomplish it. Specific training programmes are developing. There are many SHO posts in the specialty but these are mostly taken by those looking for wide experience, for training in decision-making and for career thinking-time before going off into other specialties. Few registrar and senior registrar posts exist but it is these which offer the specialty training in A & E.

In the past doctors have become senior registrars or even consultants in A & E without specific training, having a background in either medicine, surgery or anaesthetics as indicated by the MRCP, FRCS or FFA. Not only is specific training now required for specialist accreditation, but the Royal College of Surgeons of Edinburgh in partnership with the Royal College of Physicians of Edinburgh now offers an FRCS diploma in Accident and Emergency Medicine and Surgery. Candidates have to pass Part 1 of the FRCS or Part 1 of the MRCP(UK) or Part II of the FFA before they are eligible. Clinical and oral examinations include both medicine and surgery as do both short answer and multiple choice questions directed towards all aspects of medicine and surgery relating to A & E.

The work of A & E departments is a mixture of major and minor, complicated and trivial (without it always being clear initially which is which). True accidents and emergencies mingle with a large amount of minor illness which, particularly in the inner cities, gravitate to hospital rather than to general practitioners. The flow of work is often continuous and the pressure to make rapid decisions constant; with both medical and diplomatic skill the urgent has to be streamed from the not so urgent. It is a task which calls for good clinical judgement, the ability to work in a team under pressure and often with difficult or unusually demanding patients. Skill and pleasure in minor surgery is a useful attribute.

Maintenance of good communication and working relationships both with consultant and nursing colleagues and with general practitioners is essential. Patients may need to be admitted speedily with good teamwork. Most patients will be returned to the care of their general practitioners, who need to be quickly put in the picture. Good relations should be developed with the police who often bring patients in and whose help is sometimes needed to put violent intruders out. Many hospitals have a 24-hour casualty ward under the direction of the A & E consultant.

Far too many A & E consultants still work on their own without a consultant colleague to share the cover, a task hard enough for two but quite unreasonable for one. Eventually consultants may enjoy almost as good working conditions in this specialty as do their junior staff, who work on shift system already. Progress towards proper manning of A & E at all levels is slow. The A & E consultant has to combine the roles of expert in resuscitation, production-line manager and universal aunt; a challenging but enjoyable task for the right person.

Obstetrics and gynaecology (Table 8.4)

Obstetrics and gynaecology is on the one hand perhaps the most optimistic and on the other hand the most demanding specialty. Most of obstetrics and much of gynaecology concerns essentially healthy young women. Gynaecology admittedly also involves

Table 8.4. Obstetrics and gynaecology in England and Wales, 1987[2]

	Total	% Female
Consultants	793	11.6

older age groups, who have a higher incidence of serious disease, but a fatal outcome is still the exception. Most of the work is in hospital or in community outpatient clinics; obstetric flying squads add an occasional visit to patients at home.

Work patterns in obstetric training

A large amount of unpredictable emergency work at all hours is an unavoidable part of obstetrics. Stamina, resilience and a supportive and stable domestic environment are essential requirements: the first two qualities are possessed in equal measure by men and women; in the third requirement women are often but not necessarily at a disadvantage. The career is a much more realistic proposition if the spouse has work with less demanding hours, more predictable responsibilities and has a whole-hearted commitment towards his or her partner's professional fulfilment. Indeed that is a necessity if the marriage is not to be severely tried. Resilience and dedication is called for from both partners. This is very much a 'hands on' and not a contemplative specialty, requiring the attitude and practical skill of those at ease with the rewiring, plumbing and repairs, to whom practical challenges are pleasures not chores. The heavy burden of emergency work starting at SHO level, reaching a climax as registrar, continuing at a high level at senior registrar and gaining momentum as a consultant with private as well as NHS practice, ensures that this is a specialty for the addicted.

Besides the obstetrics, SHOs need to undergo an intensive and demanding period in neonatal medicine. Physically and emotionally this is one of the most demanding parts of the training. The registrar has similar duties to the SHO but more responsibility for decisions and a greater operative role, for example in undertaking caesarian sections, assuming an increasingly practical role in other approaches to complicated delivery, and obtaining experience in gynaecological surgery. There should also be an opportunity to learn techniques as varied as diagnostic ultrasound, amniocentesis and villus sampling.

The senior registrar has a more or less unsupervised operating list, a share in the senior management of deliveries and the opportunity to deputise for the consultants. Teaching of both undergraduate and postgraduate students is also an important part of the job together with prime responsibility for the day to day administration of the unit. The service load is so heavy that there is little opportunity for research unless time is deliberately taken out (see Chapter 6) or one is working in an academic unit.

The leadership of the team and final overall responsibility for the efficiency and standards of the service rests with the consultants. Hours do not diminish. Some registrars and senior registrars do not become consultants in the specialty but move sideways to become consultants in, for example, genito-urinary medicine, community medicine or family planning – all specialties with kinder hours and opportunity for part-time work compatible with family responsibilities.

Participation in abortion services is a normal part of the training and service responsibility. Clearly this may confront those with strong religious convictions with an ethical dilemma. The NHS is expected to provide abortion services and it is normal for all members of the medical team to play their part, although in exceptional circumstances different arrangements are sometimes made by agreement between colleagues.

Subspecialties in obstetrics and gynaecology

Subspecialisation starts at senior registrar level, after completion of the MRCOG, in areas such as gynaecological oncology, reproductive endocrinology, urology and urodynamics, and foetal/maternal medicine an area of interest which is well on the way to splitting into either the early antenatal period (including antenatal diagnosis of inherited disease and management of recurrent abortion) or the perinatal period including foetal monitoring.

Obstetrics and gynaecology is a very demanding and practical specialty, consuming but satisfying. Reasons for entering it range from an insatiable appetite for cliff-hanging clinical situations to the confession that 'as a man and a hypochondriac I could not get any of the diseases'.

Anaesthetics (Table 8.5)

Anaesthetics is the largest hospital specialty. A career in it starts at SHO, preferably after one or two SHO posts in other specialties. A good background in medicine with acquisition of the MRCP would seem to be highly desirable, especially for those planning to subspecialise in intensive care. Not all anaesthetic appointments committees favour a background in medicine, so it may be necessary to argue your case.

Table 8.5. Anaesthetics in England and Wales, 1987[2]

	Total	Total	% Female
Consultants	1972	2025	19.4

Work patterns in anaesthetic training

SHOs learn how to give a simple anaesthetic safely under supervision, about the problems which may arise during anaesthesia and the extent to which they can be minimised or even prevented by critical pre-operative assessment. Several practical procedures are learned at this stage including insertion of central venous lines and arterial cannulae, nerve blocks, intubation under difficult circumstances and, sometimes epidural anaesthesia, although that may be deferred to the registrar stage. There will probably be little obstetric, paediatric or pain clinic experience at this stage. An attempt is made to give the SHO a feeling of the continuity of care from pre-operative preparation through anaesthesia to early postoperative care, including analgesia and intravenous fluids. During a one-year appointment the SHO takes Part 1 and Part 2 of the FFA (see p. 60).

Anaesthetic registrars become competent to undertake routine anaesthesia unsupervised and to cope with straightforward emergencies, such as intestinal obstruction or a fractured hip. In the ITU they have greater responsibility and are expected to become proficient in performing emergency biochemical investigations including blood gas analysis and in supervising parenteral nutrition. Obstetric anaesthetic training also begins in earnest at this stage with competence quickly expected in epidural anaesthesia. While not expected to anaesthetise children under the age of one or under five if seriously ill, straightforward anaesthesia of children is involved, especially in the course of special experience in ENT, orthopaedics and accident and emergency. Experience of anaesthesia for eye surgery is also usually gained during this period. Before the end of the registrar post the final FFA must be passed because without it there is no chance of obtaining a senior registrar post.

Between registrar and senior registrar posts in this specialty is generally the most suitable moment to take one or two years out for research, for experience abroad in a good unit, for more specialised registrar experience than is part of normal rotations (for example in a specialist children's or heart hospital), for experience as a neonatal SHO to learn all aspects of neonatal care, or as a medical SHO or registrar in the case of those intending to specialise in intensive care who have not yet acquired the MRCP.

Senior registrars learn to do most things by themselves, including gaining experience now in more high-technology specialties such as neurosurgery and cardiothoracic surgery. Likewise they assume much of the responsibility for the day to day continuity of care in the ITU. Administrative responsibilities are part of the training at this level, particularly the arrangement of the duty rotas; the senior registrar also takes part in Divisional meetings.

Anaesthetic subspecialties

Consultant anaesthetists often take a special interest in one particular area such as obstetrics, cardiothoracic surgery, neurosurgery or intensive therapy unit (ITU) but they nevertheless usually retain a general commitment.

There are some part-time and some shared posts at both senior registrar and consultant level, but all posts in anaesthesia carry a heavy emergency load until the end of the consultant's career. When on duty at night the anaesthetist is likely to be working; on the other hand they sensibly try to arrange a shorter day next day.

This is a specialty for those good with their hands, people who like machines, instant doers who like to concentrate on and finish one job before going on to the next.

Psychiatric specialties (Table 8.6)

Psychiatry is steadily becoming more community-based and less confined to hospitals. Entry to the specialty is beginning to reflect this change of emphasis with more doctors now entering psychiatry from general practice Vocational Training Schemes. Others still obtain a firm grounding in general medicine first and obtain the MRCP before starting psychiatry training. Some are sufficiently sure of their career decision and single-minded in its implementation that they commence a four-year training programme in psychiatry soon after registration.

During psychiatric training leading to the MRCPsych examinations a trainee is allotted a psychiatric tutor who is expected to ensure that before taking the first part of the examination the candidate can be signed up as having completed a satisfactory training in maintenance of records and case notes, performing clinical examinations and fulfilling professional responsibilities as a member of a multidisciplinary team, besides having attended an academic course of instruction in psychiatry. Courses on a day or part-day release basis are organised at one or more centres in each region to provide an element of systematic instruction within the training programme.

Psychiatric training schemes usually comprise one year at SHO and three at registrar level, but before promotion to registrar at

Table 8.6. Psychiatry specialties in England and Wales, 1987[2]

	Consultants	
	Total	% Female
Mental illness	1251	18.0
Child and adolescent psychiatry	357	38.1
Forensic psychiatry	61	18.0
Mental handicap	171	31.0
Psychotherapy	84	22.6

the end of the first year a formal review is made of the trainee's suitability. It does seem to be in everyone's interest, not least the trainee's, that if considered unsuitable for one reason or another a change of career direction is made sooner rather than later.

Work patterns in psychiatric training

The SHO is part of a clinical team and has outpatient, day-patient and inpatient responsibilities. Only the most seriously disturbed patients are admitted to hospital and as there are no preregistration house officers in psychiatry the SHO is responsible for coordinating investigation and treatment often involving several disciplines, besides making day to day or even hour to hour adjustments in drug treatment. Night duty for both emergency admissions and problems on the wards is likely to be about once a week. The SHO's work is supervised by a senior registrar who is also responsible for much of the teaching.

The registrar's duties are similar to those of the SHO but with more responsibility and less supervision. Rotations are usually arranged through all major areas of psychiatry, including adult, child, forensic and liaison psychiatry, psychotherapy, rehabilitation and mental handicap. Part 2 of the MRCPsych is taken during the registrar period. There is no chance of a senior registrar post without the MRCPsych and the sooner it is obtained the better the prospect of obtaining one of the most sought-after senior registrar or lecturer posts.

Subspecialisation in psychiatry

Some senior registrar posts are entirely subspecialty based, for example in child or forensic psychiatry, psychogeriatrics or mental handicap, or they pass through several general and specialist posts, with a predominant period in adult psychiatry and one particular subspecialty which will result in accreditation as a general adult psychiatrist with a declared special interest. Elective sessions are given to enable gaps in specialty experience to be filled and two sessions should be provided throughout the senior registrar training for research and private study. There are few opportunities for long periods in research but up to one year can be counted as part of accredited training.

Psychiatry is a very clinical discipline. It is unusual in that more than any other specialty it has to balance the needs of patients against the needs of society, indeed the psychiatrist is the one doctor in a position directly to deny a patient his liberty. A facility for listening and an interest in how people 'tick' is necessary. An ability to work as a member of a largely nonmedical, multi-disciplinary team is essential. Consultant psychiatrists in the NHS are entitled to retire at the age of 55 on full pension provided they have at least 20 years of continuous service, a reflection of the perception that working with the mentally ill is particularly stressful.

9

Clinical support services

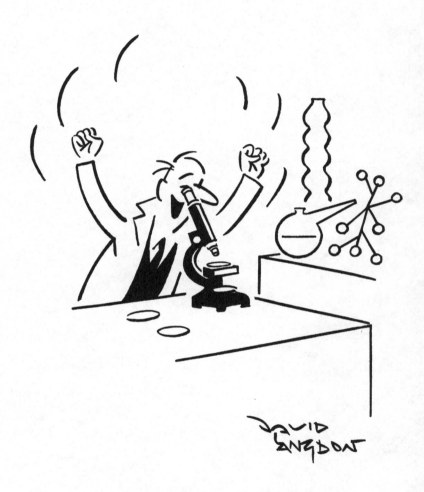

. . . enjoy looking down a microscope . . .

9
Clinical support services

Pathology specialties (Table 9.1)

While there is something in common between the pathology
specialties the precise nature of the work of each is different. They
all provide diagnostic laboratory services, each specialty examining a different aspect of pathological processes and the light
which they throw on the diagnosis of disease, its treatment and
prevention. Pathologists need to have a practical working knowledge of the tests which they interpret and of the disease conditions
to which they relate. They need to be able to vouch for the
accuracy of the tests their laboratory provides by continuous
monitoring of quality control. They have to be able to communicate their opinion succinctly, verbally and in writing, to colleagues in both hospital and general practice. Laboratory
management also becomes an important part of their skills and
they need more than a passing knowledge of the process of
computerisation of test results and records.

Some pathologists, especially haematologists but also some
medical microbiologists, chemical pathologists and immunologists, take responsibility for clinical care as well as for their
laboratory investigation. The widely varying balance of laboratory work and clinical responsibility between and within different
branches of pathology in different locations, the intrinsic scientific base of each discipline, the element of detective work and

129

their relatively well-ordered lifestyle make these specialties attractive to those who look discerningly at them.

The training programmes are based on apprentice-type education which until recently had both a degree of integration and a common pattern; in future only the pattern will be similar. Whereas both the early part of training and the first examination provided and tested, respectively, a wide background of pathology, the training will in future be restricted to one branch. Both Part 1 and Part 2 of the new examinations for Membership of the Royal College of Pathologists (MRCPath) will be single-specialty-based and will not include multidisciplinary questions. It is for the pathologists to decide if this narrower approach is educationally desirable but from the point of view of men and women who wish to sample before deciding, or having decided, wish after a year or two to change their minds, the change seems retrogressive. The special knowledge and skill required in each branch remains the same, bearing in mind that each specialty is evolving rapidly in its techniques and is continuing to make new demands and to give new opportunities to its proponents.

A broad critical training in pathology will always remain educational and useful. Clinical experience also must surely widen perspectives and improve the ability to communicate with colleagues, while for those hoping to combine laboratory work with clinical responsibility an appropriate clinical training is essential.

Management skills are required of consultants in all branches of pathology. To direct a department successfully it is necessary to be interested in all grades of staff, to mix easily with them and to

Table 9.1. Pathology specialties in England and Wales, 1987[2]

	Consultants	
	Total	% Female
Histopathology	599	21.2
Neuropathology	29	24.1
Immunopathology	40	12.5
Medical microbiology	322	24.5
Haematology	380	21.8
Blood transfusion	33	24.2
Chemical pathology	203	12.3

be sympathetic to their requirements for in-service training and career advancement. Good financial management and an interest in the economics of the health service is also demanded of budget-holders.

Histopathology and related specialties

Histopathologists are no longer merely or mainly archivists of death and cataloguers of surgical specimens. Many of the specimens they now examine are needle or endoscopic biopsies. Their examinations of tissues have become multidimensional reconstructions of the nature of the underlying disease process, describing not just appearances by light and electron microscope but processes revealed by a whole range of new histochemical, immunocytochemical and molecular biological techniques.

Although possession of the MRCP or FRCS will no longer give exemption from Part 1 of the MRCPath examination, the value of a wide clinical background in relating histological appearances to clinical consequences is surely as great as ever. Narrower training may magnify the detail but blur the context. A year or two in medical or surgical SHO posts and in at least one other branch of pathology gives an excellent if not now an essential foundation to a career in pathology.

Receiving and describing operative or needle biopsy specimens and indicating how they are to be sectioned and stained is a substantial part of a histopathology registrar's apprenticeship. Preliminary reporting follows, but the final report is made by or in conjunction with a consultant. Likewise, frozen sections have to be prepared ready for consultant reporting. Postmortem examinations (necropsies) are part of the task with presentation of the findings at case conferences and clinical meetings. Technical expertise has to be acquired especially in newer techniques; a minimum of three months must be spent in cytology and one month in a sub-specialty such as neuropathology.

Currently it is necessary to pass the primary examination for the MRCPath before starting higher training as a senior registrar. It is not yet clear where the new Part 1 examination will fit into the professional pathway, whether between registrar and senior registrar, as now, or early in the senior registrar period. Progression to senior registrar is facilitated by publications which are usually based on service work. Only in academic units is there a substantial opportunity for experimental research. Senior registrars may in addition to their routine work be asked to perform postmortem examinations for the coroner, and to present the findings at the coroner's court. Forensic pathology itself is a separate training offered in only a few academic departments. Senior registrars also learn laboratory management and participate in various District committees. Management skills are important, especially if hospital laboratory staff remain as they were once described in blanket fashion, 'an underpaid and chronically dissatisfied workforce'.

Contrary to the traditional view of histopathologists as remote figures living in an atmosphere of death, dust and formalin, much of their work involves a lively interaction with clinicians. To be successful they need to communicate and to advise well; to be fulfilled they need to be fascinated by the pathological basis of disease, interested in cells and tissues, and to enjoy looking down a microscope. An analytical approach is required but can be learned. The hours are predictable; few of the tasks have to be undertaken at specific times, apart from frozen sections and clinical meetings. Part-time training is entirely feasible but it is preferable to pass Part 1 of the MRCPath first. This is a specialty which could perfectly well lend itself to shared posts.

Immunopathology, immunology and clinical immunology

Immunopathology, immunology and clinical immunology are all aspects of the one discipline concerned with the role of immunological reactions in the prevention, causation and diagnosis of disease. It is a relatively small discipline in the NHS but many universities have departments of immunology, some of which have medical interests.

Immunological techniques are used in all branches of pathology both as diagnostic tools in infective, biochemical, neoplastic and haematological diseases and in the diagnosis and monitoring of diseases caused by malfunction of the immune system itself. Diagnostic tests are variously directed towards the detection of autoantibodies to tissues or individual cell components or towards infective agents.

Clinical immunologists are particularly likely to be involved with the care of patients with antibody-induced disease (including tissue rejection after transplantation) or with failure of the immune system to prevent infective disease, as with HIV infection. They may also or alternatively work clinically in the field of allergic diseases such as asthma, hay fever and insect stings.

Entry to training in clinical immunology is usually at senior registrar level. There are few posts and even fewer as registrar. Until that point appropriate training includes a good clinical training, acquisition of the MRCP and a good grounding in laboratory techniques, usually in conjunction with a period of research for a higher degree.

Medical microbiology, including virology

Medical microbiologists are involved in a wide range of clinical practice inside and outside hospital. Their work takes them into every department and facility of the hospital. Not only is diagnosis a prime task but so also is prevention and treatment, especially advice about choice of antibiotic in the light of the nature and specific *in vitro* sensitivities and assessment of their effectiveness, including measurement of blood levels. Part of the attraction of microbiology lies in the challenge of keeping one step ahead of organisms with the ability to change and the excitement of discovering new pathogens.

Infections have contributed much of the historical drama of disease and medical microbiology continues to have a high public profile. A clinical advisory role is an integral part of the job of a consultant medical microbiologist, for example in the diagnosis and treatment of infectious disease, in control of infection in hospital wards and in prevention of disease both personally by immunisation and institutionally by kitchen inspections and checks on air conditioning systems. Of all the medical staff the medical microbiologist is the one most conversant with what is in the corners and under the carpets of the hospital. If working in the Public Health Laboratory Service this knowledge will extend into the surrounding community.

One or two general SHO posts should precede entry into medical microbiology, preferably including at least six months on an infectious diseases unit. The first year or two in the specialty is spent learning basic techniques used for examining each type of specimen, including Gram stains, plating, microscopy and setting up serological assays. There is little or no service responsibility at first, only the chance to learn, including an opportunity to understudy the more senior medical microbiologists in the other two major areas of their activity, control of infection and consulting on ward patients.

Later the registrar becomes a useful pair of hands in the laboratory (including often sharing weekend on-call duties with the MLSOs) and participates in improving day to day techniques. While lacking sufficient experience to interpret the significance of bacterial cultures there is an opportunity to attend the reporting and to discuss interpretations and advice to be given. Time is also spent taking specimens and assisting in control of infection duties. Visits are made to the central sterilising facility. A half-day release course provides systematic instruction for the first part of the MRCPath. There should also be an opportunity to undertake a laboratory-based project.

Senior registrars have a full service responsibility, reviewing cultures, signing the diagnostic reports, visiting problem patients and discussing their management with clinicians, answering telephone queries about choice of antibiotic treatment or about the degree of isolation necessary for patients suffering from known infections or undiagnosed fevers. Specimens have to be sent off with covering letters to reference laboratories. Control of infection problems have to be discussed with the control of infection senior nurse, running statistics have to be kept and reports have to be prepared for the control of infection meeting. The Medical Officer of Environmental Health has to be given early warning about any possible cases of notifiable disease.

The consultant takes an overview of all these activities in both a training and a chief of service capacity, while managing the laboratory and pursuing special interests in laboratory research or administration.

Virology has a separate training programme, at least from the senior registrar stage. There are few senior registrar posts and even fewer registrars in virology. Cell culture and electron microscopy are two techniques basic to virologists but rarely used by bacteriologists. There are hardly any virology posts in the NHS,

posts being either in university departments or in the Public
Health Laboratory Service (PHLS). The PHLS offers an alternative training programme and career opportunity to medical microbiologists. Its laboratories form a nationwide network, mostly
situated in hospitals and often providing both the hospital service
and a service to general practitioners. They also serve the environmental health services and include in that responsibility analysis
of water, food and milk and a participating role in the investigation of outbreaks of disease, such as legionnaires disease, in the
community. Doctors working for the PHLS are more directed in
what they do and where they work than those in the NHS but are
better provided for in equipment and accommodation.

To be a successful medical microbiologist it is necessary to be
scrupulously attentive to detail, to have a detective instinct, to be
patient in awaiting results, to have a wide interest in medicine, to
have up-to-date knowledge of the world geography of pathogens
and to be a good communicator with colleagues to the point of
being able to impose by agreement unpalatable measures such as
the closure of wards and operating theatres on grounds of risk of
infection.

Haematology

Haematology combines laboratory investigation with clinical
care, a combination which not only explains its popularity but
also its demanding training. In addition to providing laboratory
investigation of any blood disorder the haematology service
usually also runs the blood transfusion laboratory. Not all
patients with blood diseases come under the care of haematologists but the complicated ones, including haemophiliacs,
patients with aplastic anaemias, myelofibrosis, haemoglobino-
pathies, bleeding disorders, lymphomas and leukaemias usually
do and are likely to benefit from this specialist care. Haematologists also usually mount an anticoagulant clinic.

The demands of the job are such that it is necessary to have a
training in medicine to MRCP standard and in haematology to
MRCPath; that is a formidable and lengthy undertaking.
Normally the MRCP is taken first, usually from an SHO post in
general medicine but it is sometimes taken from a haematology
post.

A registrar in haematology combines clinical liaison work, arising either from abnormalities noticed on routine report forms or from calls from clinicians for advice, with personal care of patients with haematological conditions both as inpatients and in outpatient clinics. At the same time, or in periods in the laboratory alternating with periods on clinical service, the registrar has to become proficient in a wide variety of standard laboratory techniques. These include the examination of blood films and bone marrow, performing coagulation tests, investigations of haemolytic and other anaemias, testing for antibodies to red cells, using isotopic methods for labelling red cells *in vivo* and determination of blood groups and crossmatching for transfusion. Clinical techniques to be learned include bone marrow aspiration and trephine biopsy in addition to all the usual practical procedures of general medicine, not least the repeated transfusion of patients with few remaining accessible veins. The diagnosis and care of patients with leukaemia, myeloma and lymphoma together with administration of chemotherapy is another of the clinical responsibilities. Bone marrow transplantation is a further dimension at some centres.

The senior registrar has similar tasks but at a more supervisory level and with greater personal clinical responsibility including acting for the consultant in laboratory and ward. Teaching undergraduates, postgraduates and technical staff occupies part of the time. Laboratory management is learned at this stage partly by apprenticeship and partly by participating in the administrative structure of the hospital and Health District. At least three months must be spent in a transfusion centre and a total of at least six months training in transfusion techniques, preparation of blood, testing for hepatitis, HIV and other hazards. A minority of consultants work purely in blood transfusion (see Table 9.1).

Chemical pathology (clinical chemistry, clinical biochemistry)

The different names adopted by those who provide and advise clinicians on the selection and interpretation of biochemical tests indicate the widely different emphasis adopted by departments. Departments range from the nonclinically-led with little clinical involvement to those directed by a clinical biochemist who combines some duties of a metabolic physician with running the diagnostic service. In many places the biochemical diagnostic service is regarded as entirely a part of the pathology services; in a few this service, while no less rigorously scientific, is an integral part of metabolic medicine. The important thing is to have a first rate, rapid, reliable diagnostic service and readily available informed advice. Administrative structures should be moulded to local circumstances so as best to achieve this. Either way, there is also a responsibility to teach medical and laboratory staff in chemical pathology/clinical biochemistry and often, undergraduate medical students too.

Training in this as in the other pathology sub-specialties is becoming narrower but it stands to reason that if a department is to have a large role in advising clinical staff, if not actually running metabolic clinics and a metabolic investigation ward, the medical staff in the specialty need to have a solid clinical grounding and experience besides their biochemical expertise. For this reason sufficient clinical experience to acquire the MRCP before entering chemical pathology has much to recommend it. Such a background leaves a biochemical gap to be filled either by taking an MSc, often on day-release in-service training, or by taking time out to acquire a PhD, or by having taken a biochemistry degree before entering medicine as a mature student.

Registrars in the specialty are expected to become competent technically in all standard analyses such as flame spectrophotometry, electrophoresis, chromatography and immunoassay, so as to be conversant with them and with their underlying principles. Quality control of methods and a facility in computerisation for reporting results rapidly within hospital and outside and of storing records are other important aspects. Other duties include signing and commenting on report forms, answering telephone queries from hospital staff and general practitioners and participating in clinical meetings. In some hospitals, suitably qualified and experienced registrars in chemical pathology participate in diabetic and endocrine clinics.

While as a registrar there should be an opportunity to undertake some original research; senior registrars are currently required to present a laboratory-based research project as part of the final MRCPath and this will continue to be an option in the new Part 2. The day to day analytical work is competently under-

taken by biochemists and MLSOs but there is still a need to be
fully conversant with the methods used and the problems which
may arise with them, besides taking initiatives in the evaluation
and introduction of alternative methods. In routine diagnostic
departments research is usually based on everyday opportunity
and need. Higher degrees are not usually obtained by the medical
staff except by those in university departments.

Managerial skills are learned as a senior registrar. Possibly
greater managerial skill is called for in chemical pathology than in
other branches of pathology because of its three-stranded administration: the MLSOs are responsible to the senior chief MLSO;
biochemists to the top-grade biochemist; medical staff to the
consultant chemical pathologist, who is also normally the director of department, budget-holder and in overall charge. Inter-
disciplinary rivalries have sometimes marred the harmony of
departments and considerable managerial skill is required.

On-call duties for medical staff in this discipline are not heavy
and can be undertaken from home. It is a suitable specialty for
those with domestic commitments.

Diagnostic radiology and radiotherapy (Table 9.2)

Diagnostic radiology

Diagnostic radiology is almost as large a specialty as general
medicine. It is a specialty full of diagnostic interest, which has
substantial involvement with both patients and clinicians without
the ties of continuing responsibility for the care of patients. The
imaging technologies available have advanced rapidly, giving

Table 9.2. Diagnostic Radiology and Radiotherapy in England
and Wales, 1987[2]

	Consultants	
	Total	% Female
Diagnostic radiology	1042	20.0
Nuclear medicine	27	18.5
Radiotherapy	216	16.7

immediate access to parts of the body no previous techniques have reached as easily or effectively. Advances in instrumentation have increased the opportunity for the employment of practical skills in diagnosis and in treatment by interventional radiology. Interpretation of images requires a wide background knowledge of diagnostic possibilities which can only effectively be obtained by clinical experience before entering the discipline. The Royal College of Radiologists insists on at least one year of postregistration experience, preferably clinical, before embarking on training in diagnostic radiology. Many enter the specialty after obtaining the MRCP, some the FRCS.

Training schemes are based on university hospitals or large District General Hospitals and involve rotation to either or both specialist postgraduate hospitals and smaller District General Hospitals. Two or three years are spent as a registrar with attendance at a formal half-day release course during university terms.

The sudden demotion in responsibility in the first year of training is generally a shock to those entering the specialty as SHOs who have already been registrars in another discipline and have obtained a higher diploma in that clinical specialty. Further, there is initially no on-call commitment and the salary is therefore less than in clinical posts. A simultaneous fall in both responsibility and income is not good for self respect. There is inevitably an initial period of observing but before long an SHO and certainly a registrar undertakes standard fluoroscopic examinations such as barium studies. Also there is reporting to be done, but all reports are checked by a more senior member of the department until Part 1 of the FRCR has been passed. Most interventional procedures are learned later. It is a difficult transition period but there is no reason at all to be disheartened – there are better times ahead. The important thing is to be prepared for the transition.

Many training schemes require trainees to pass Part 1 at first or second attempt, i.e. in the first year of the scheme, if they are to continue. The interest steadily increases. More responsibility is given in reporting; techniques such as angiography, myelography, computerised tomography and ultrasound are introduced, scanning-directed needle biopsies and nephrostomies are undertaken, on-call duties (mainly for emergency scanning and some interventional work such as nephrostomies and angiography) begin again. Administrative tasks such as arranging duty rotas are also a part of the responsibility.

Depending on the department and on competition at the time, the final FRCR may or may not be expected before obtaining a senior registrar post today. With increasing competition and more interchange between training schemes the FRCR may soon be required to obtain any senior registrar post. Senior registrars play a large part in the everyday work of a department but they also have an opportunity to develop a special interest in a sub-specialty such as interventional radiology, scanning or clinical physics/nuclear medicine, often with a year abroad at a special centre, usually now in the USA where radiological technology is further advanced overall than in the UK.

Radiology is very much a practically-based service specialty in which research has not been a large element. Publications are expected but are usually very clinically-based, arising out of everyday routine work. Higher degrees are not expected of consultants, other than in academic units. Teaching trainee radiologists and radiographers, also often medical students, is a usual responsibility. Accreditation is acquired after five years in the specialty and a consultant post is usually obtained soon afterwards.

Radiotherapy

History but little else seems to make sense of the bracketing of the specialties of radiotherapy and diagnostic radiology. Ionising radiations were found to have both diagnostic and therapeutic uses and there perhaps the commonalty ends.

Radiotherapy is concerned with the calculation and delivery of therapeutic or palliative doses of ionising radiations, usually to patients with cancer but also occasionally to those with other conditions. Radiotherapy departments were previously often responsible for diagnostic clinical physics but the medical direction of that area now usually falls to the radiologists or to consultants in nuclear medicine. In so far as the technical aspects of calculation of dosage and its delivery are concerned, physicists might be considered to be more appropriate than doctors. The real art is in deciding the indications for this form of treatment in relation to alternatives such as surgery or, more commonly, chemotherapy. The lead here has on the whole been taken by medical oncologists not by radiotherapists and it becomes increasingly apparent that the care of the patient, the diagnosis and assessment of optimum therapy, its delivery and the patient's follow-up should all be in the hands of one joint team.

Expert advice should be taken on the pathway of training in this changing field. A unit which offers a combined training in medical oncology and radiotherapy would seem to be best, with the opportunity as senior registrar level to steer more towards one aspect than the other while retaining general competence.

For radiotherapy itself, a background training in general medicine is highly desirable, including a period in medical oncology. Acquisition of the MRCP is a good investment. While undertaking a radiotherapy registrar post, in which instruction is given in the requisite physics, the handling of isotopes and techniques of radiotherapy, the Part 1 of the FRCR should be obtained. Part 2 is usually obtained while undergoing apprenticeship training in service as a senior registrar. Clinical work is mainly on an outpatient basis. Research opportunities purely in radiotherapy are not great and higher degrees are not necessary in order to secure a consultant post. The specialty involves regular hours.

Medical administration

Doctors have the medical knowledge of the nature of the service, the commitment to providing a first-class service and the necessary understanding of people to become good managers of health services despite the lack of any formal training. Not all have the necessary flair and interest but many have. Doctors have long had a key managerial role in public health in which they have set a framework for action, turning circumstances and regulations into prescriptions for action. General practitioners have long had to attend to the business management of their practices. In hospitals doctors used to have a key managerial role but it has been unfashionable for several decades. Formerly a medical superintendent was a normal part of the managerial structure and that is still so in the USA and Australasia, where a medical administrator, trained professionally for the purpose, either manages medical services and staff or serves as director of the whole hospital.

A few doctors in Britain today become full-time health service managers in competition with professional administrators, but there is no formal training or career structure. All this may rapidly change and a Cinderella specialty may become a mainline career opportunity within a few years. Clinical resource management is a different and rapidly evolving function of a larger number of hospital doctors.

All doctors in NHS hospitals are increasingly being held responsible to some degree for the resources they deploy. Some have already taken responsibility for a budget for their own particular service. In other hospitals medical staff have accepted a global budget for each specialty and appointed one of themselves as doctor manager/financial director for each. In that capacity, the medical manager (assisted by a full-time NHS administrator) has to consider the most effective work patterns of consultants and junior staff, measures to reduce waiting lists, prescribing policies and other aspects of running an excellent and cost-effective service. Clinical responsibility and choice of treatment remain the prerogative of the individual consultant but he no longer makes decisions in splendid isolation. A new sense of purpose, cohesion, quality and cost-effectiveness seems to have been achieved by hospitals which have taken this road to medical management. The burden on clinicians, most of whom would prefer to give all their energy to their clinical work, is considerable but the general view seems to be that this is the pattern for the future.

Medical services have probably suffered in the past from doctors looking at management and financial accountability as matters for others. Only recently has the need become recognised in the profession to second some of the best trained, most able and well organised doctors to steer the ships that make the navy.

Careers are also available in health service administration at the Department of Health. These are concerned with matters such as manpower planning, national policies on audit, public health and health education. A few posts are also available for doctors in the administration of medical research charities.

IO

Public health/community medicine and occupational health

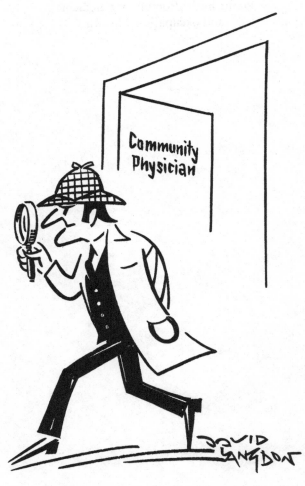

... keen observation and good detective work ...

10

Public health/community medicine and occupational health

Public health/community medicine (Table 10.1)

Table 10.1. Senior community medicine staff in England and Wales, 1987[2]

Total	Regional medical officers	District medical officers	Specialists in community medicine
494	11	140	343

Keen observation and good detective work have been at the heart of the development of public health, and interest in public health has done much to encourage keen observation and good detective work. John Snow is an outstanding example. He was not in fact a public health doctor either by occupation or background, indeed his reputation rested on being one of the first doctors to administer anaesthetics in clinical practice, including to Queen Victoria herself. But it was impossible to live and work in London in the mid-nineteenth century without being concerned about cholera. Snow noticed one crucial difference between the cholera epidemic of 1849 and those of 1853 and 1854. In all three years, areas dependent on the Thames River for their water supply, whether by pail or by pipe, were particularly badly hit, but some of those areas badly affected in 1849 were strikingly spared in 1853 and 1854.

Most of these areas were south of the river and were supplied either entirely by the Southwark and Vauxhall Water Company, entirely by the Lambeth Water Company or by both. Snow discovered through an analysis of deaths reported to the General Registrar's Office and from the water company records that those parishes supplied by Lambeth, which had suffered badly in 1849, had a much reduced mortality in 1853 and 1854, while those supplied by Southwark and Vauxhall suffered equally badly throughout. In 1849 both companies drew their water from the Thames in central London but in 1852 the Lambeth Company started piping water from the rural district of Thames Ditton well upstream and ceased taking water from central London. In the 1854 outbreak mortality from cholera, which had been similar in the areas supplied by both companies in 1849, was five times higher in areas supplied by the Southwark and Vauxhall Company.

Snow saw that the real test of the hypothesis that cholera was caused by a chemical or biological waterborne agent in water polluted by the excreta of sufferers from the disease, lay in those areas supplied jointly by the two companies because

> ... the mixing of supply is of the most intimate kind. The pipes of each company go down all the streets, and into nearly all the courts and alleys ... As there is no difference whatever, either in the houses or the people receiving the supply of the water companies, or in any of the physical conditions with which they are surrounded, it is obvious that no experiment could have been devised which would more thoroughly test the effect of water supply on the progress of cholera.
>
> The experiment was on the grandest scale. No fewer than 300,000 people of both sexes, of every age and occupation, and of every rank and station, from gentlefolk down to the very poor, were divided into two groups without their choice, and in most cases without their knowledge, one group being supplied with water containing the sewerage of London and, amongst it whatever might have come from cholera patients, the other having water quite free from such impurity.

Amongst this jumble of water pipes 266 516 people were supplied by Southwark and Vauxhall in 1854, and 4093 died of cholera (153 per 10 000); 173 748 were supplied by Lambeth, and 461 died (26 per 10 000).

The evidence was strong but circumstantial; the causative agent could not be identified and there were other difficulties, such as the explosive outbreak at Broad Street remote from Thames water but clustered around another water supply, the Broad Street pump in Golden Square. In the last week of August in 1854 amongst those living around Broad Street, 4 died in the first 4 days, 4 died on the fifth day and over the weekend 79 people died, mostly within 24 hours of first developing symptoms. All but 10 lived close to the pump and of these exceptions, 5 always obtained their water from the Broad Street pump 'because they preferred it' and 3 more were children who went to school nearby and drank from the pump.

There were several inconsistencies but they all proved to have convincing explanations: for example, there were no cases amongst workers in the percussion cap factory in Broad Street (which turned out to have its own well) nor in the brewery ('The men are allowed to drink a certain quantity of malt liquour and Mr. Huggins believes they do not drink water at all'; in any event the brewery had its own water supply); and only 5 cases occurred in the workhouse which, if it had been affected in proportion to the rest of the district, would have had over 100 cases. That too had its own water supply.

How the water become contaminated was never established but the pump handle was removed a few days later by order of the Parish Council and the outbreak subsided. Snow could not explain why many people apparently exposed to infected water did *not* develop the disease but that paradox applied to many other apparently communicable diseases. Although both the reason for getting and for not getting cholera was unknown that did not prevent observations leading to prevention.

The intriguing and immensely rewarding challenge of the identification by epidemiological means of the source, cause and means of prevention of disease, whether legionnaires disease or coronary artery disease, continues chameleon-like to assume new colours, but it is only one dimension of public health.

The specialty of public health arose out of the social reforms of the nineteenth century. The Medical Officers of Health (MOH) appointed by and responsible to each local authority have played a key role. As social conditions improved and infectious diseases declined the importance of the MOH diminished, the role changed and, in 1974, the name became Community Physician. Now Regional and District Medical Officers have become Regional and District Directors of Public Health, respectively, and Specialists in Community Medicine have become Consultants in Public Health Medicine. About the same time, academic departments of Epidemiology or Community Medicine sprang up in many universities, rightly establishing epidemiology as the scientific foundation of public health. Epidemiology is directed particularly towards the identification of causes of disease. Public health is also concerned with the 'analysis of health needs of particular population groups (such as the homeless and ethnic minorities) and with the provision, organisation and evaluation of services'.[25] Preventive medicine and health education are other dimensions.

The Acheson Report on *Public Health in England*[25] envisages a new dimension of leadership by doctors in public health and a new sense of direction in its programmes of postgraduate education. This new-style approach to public health has the opportunity to be at the centre of the development of health services in Britain, providing the mixture of medicine and politics on which health services depend. The emphasis is on a global view of health care and on the critical evaluation of health policy and its outcome. Training for public health is underpinned by the philosophy in the Report that 'no health service can sensibly operate without disease prevention and health promotion and without evaluating outcome' and that public health is 'the science and art of preventing disease, prolonging life and promoting health through organised efforts of society'. District Directors of Public Health will be deeply involved in the objective assessment and evaluation of existing services and their improvement; they will be required to report annually on their progress in achieving the following responsibilities:

1. To review regularly the health of the population for which they are responsible and to identify problems. To define objectives and to set targets to deal with the problems in the light of national and regional guidelines.

2. To relate the decisions which they take about the investment of resources to their impact on the health problems and objectives so identified.
3. To evaluate progress towards their stated objectives.
4. To make arrangements for the surveillance, prevention, treatment and control of communicable disease and infection.
5. To give advice to and seek cooperation with other agencies and organisations in the locality to promote health.

Directors at Regional level will also be expected

to make plans for dealing with major outbreaks of communicable disease and infection which span more than one district and ensure their implementation.

Achieving and maintaining closer liaison between District Health Authorities, family practitioners and local authorities, including with the local authority's Chief Environmental Officer (the local authority's main source of advice on environmental health issues) is a large task. A District Control of Infection Officer (DCIO) who will be a member of the District Department of Public Health and responsible to its director, will have executive responsibility for action to control communicable disease. The DCIO may either work fulltime in public health or combine DCIO responsibility with that of a consultant in another specialty such as infectious diseases or microbiology. Provision of public information on outbreaks of infection and on routine issues of control and prevention of communicable disease is part of the brief. The specialty is expanding, and training opportunities are good. A resurgence of interest in public health complements and should encourage parallel development of the sub-specialty of infectious diseases, including sexually transmitted diseases (genitourinary medicine). Related career opportunities are to be found in the Public Health Laboratory Service (most appropriately for those with a microbiological background training) and in the Communicable Diseases Surveillance Centre (for which epidemiology might be the best background).

Intending applicants should seek the advice of Regional Faculty Advisers or Regional District Directors of Public Health or a Professor of Community Medicine/Public Health. Coordination of the postgraduate training and most of the training posts themselves will be in the hands of Regional Health Authorities, but the overall objectives, higher diploma regulations and continuing

education requirements are likely to continue to be determined by
the Faculty of Community Medicine of the Royal Colleges of
Physicians of the United Kingdom.

Occupational health

Occupational medicine is a mixture of preventive and rather
administrative general medicine; it covers a wide range of activities designed to protect the health and welfare of people at work.
A broad general professional training is required in clinical SHO
posts, either all in hospital specialties or on a general practice
Vocational Training Scheme to gain a broader perspective and
wider experience. An MSc in clinical epidemiology would be a
good basis for understanding the investigative aspects of occupational medicine. Towards the end of a three year period of
postregistration general professional training a post should be
obtained in occupational medicine and work should begin on a
part-time or fulltime academic course in the principles of the
subject leading up to acquisition of the diploma of Associate of
the Faculty of Occupational Medicine (AFOM).

A few training posts are available in academic departments, but
both posts and departments are few. Most of the posts suitable for
training are in industry, some of them being joint posts between a
university and an industrial department. Only large firms have a
medically led occupational health service sufficiently large to be
able to provide training posts; training may be full- or part-time.
Smaller firms tend not to have their own employed medical staff
but to take medical advice on a consultancy basis.

The work itself is partly desk work, partly overseeing the
Clinical Occupational Health Service in the workplace, which is
normally run by occupational health-trained nurses, and partly a
matter of being out and about in the factory or industry so as to
understand the nature of the health hazards, meet staff and investigate particular problems.

In any place of work there are general problems of personal
health, happiness and lifestyle which affect individual ability to
do a good day's work. Poor attendance records have to be investigated, possible explanations such as alcoholism have to be

considered and measures to solve such problems discussed with the individuals concerned and with management. The doctor is in a different relationship to the employee from the usual doctor–patient relationship. In this situation the doctor is responsible to his employer although clearly concerned for the welfare of the employee too. The occupational health physician is not responsible for the clinical care of individuals, other than in emergencies at work, for the employee remains the patient of his general practitioner. ·

A substantial part of the work, which depends in detail on the nature of the industry, concerns surveillance of health at work, of accidents and accident prevention, and of possible hazards arising from toxic processes or, indeed, the institutional environment with respect for example to air conditioning and the risk of *Legionella* infection.

Industrial legislation, its impact on working conditions and on compensation for any possible injuries at work must be familiar to the doctor. He may well have to consider representations from trades unions concerning conditions in general or specific cases. In his ability to communicate with, gain the confidence of and reassure the unions and employees themselves concerning health and welfare at work, the occupational health physician can contribute a great deal to the morale of a workforce. His or her expertise can also help to obtain fair compensation for disease or injury arising from work, ensure any possible rehabilitation and also provide advice and help in negotiating a change in the nature of employment within the organisation when necessary on health grounds.

The occupational health physician is in a unique position as health broker between management and employees; he or she should be a mine of information and a tower of strength to both parties. There will always be opportunities for research in this field, not least in discovering new hazards of industrial processes or methods of work, but the facilities for research are not likely to be good except in the largest organisations. A thesis based on original work done normally while undertaking supervised training in the discipline is one of the requirements for the AFOM examination, which is taken during four years of specialist training. The supervised training (and the subject of the thesis) have to be approved by the Faculty of Occupational Medicine. The train-

ing posts must be approved by the JCHMT if accreditation as a
specialist is to be gained.

Occupational medicine offers regular hours and good opportunity for part-time work. It may be combined with other work,
such as general practice, or may be a fulltime commitment in large
private or state industries, the universities, the NHS, and in the
Health and Safety Executive or its Employment Medical Advisory
Service. This is an expanding specialty which offers a wide variety
of work requiring skills in communication and administration, an
understanding of industrial processes and working practices and
lively clinical acumen.

II

Science, industry, the Armed
Services, journalism and other
careers

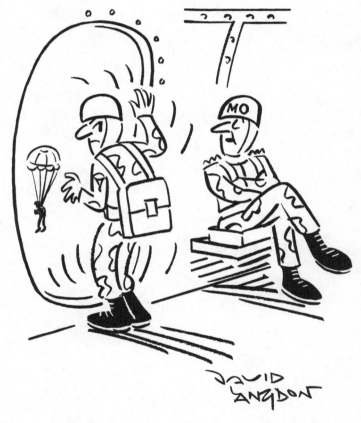

'It's called vertigo in the trade ...'

11

Science, industry, the Armed Services, journalism and other careers

Basic medical science

A few medical graduates find their way into nonmedical science departments in universities or industry, their medical training being more or less incidental to their final career. Some highly accomplished scientists take a medical degree to assist them in directing their scientific skills to medical research. Good opportunities exist for medical graduates in basic medical science departments teaching medical and, often, sciences students, and researching across the borders between basic science and clinical medicine. Basic medical science departments have a heavy teaching load but are as productive in their scientific research as any other academic department.

Medically qualified applicants have an edge in obtaining posts in basic medical science departments because it is easier for them to highlight the clinical relevance which especially interests medical students. Most departments would, however, rather recruit first class scientists who are not medical graduates than second rate scientists who are. For many years, posts in the basic medical sciences have not attracted many medical graduates, partly because clinical salaries are higher and partly because most medical graduates want to be clinicians, even if continuing in research as scientists in the clinical sciences. Anatomy, biochemistry, physiology and pharmacology all offer excellent opportunities but competition from nonmedical scientists is now intense.

Industry

The pharmaceutical industry employs medical graduates as research scientists (although most of their research scientists are not medically trained), as clinical research directors or advisers, and sometimes, they go on to become senior managers. Posts in industry are better paid than in the NHS or universities but are generally less secure. They are demanding but the supporting resources are good. Clinical research posts generally involve a considerable amount of travel, organising trials of new treatments and participating in postgraduate meetings.

The Armed Services

The Armed Forces are a world of their own; you either like Service life or you do not. For those at home in a relatively regimented structure, more stereotyped than the also somewhat hierarchical and traditional civilian medical profession, and prepared to commit themselves to several years of contracted employment, the Armed Forces offer doctors an attractive proposition. Work is assured for several years after qualification and any loss of freedom of choice is offset by security and continuity of employment together with the financial consequences of moving around the country, or the world, taken care of. Financial costs are not the only costs of moving around but the disruption is cushioned for those whose wives and families enjoy the comradeship of service life. A well structured scheme of postgraduate training is another advantage. Salaries are at least as good as in the NHS and hidden benefits, of which there are few in the NHS, are substantial.

Duties include being prepared to provide acute medical services under battle conditions, skills useful also in Civil Defence. Training nonmedical support staff, who are very much in the front line in time of war, is a continuing task. General practitioner services are the main area of medical activity of doctors in the armed forces, both in permanent bases and in support of units on active service; preventive medicine and a knowledge of disease worldwide figure larger in their work than they do for general practitioners in civilian practice. Most Service doctors work in the UK but there are still medical posts in bases in Germany and the Far East. Overseas postings also include periods at sea for medical officers in the Royal Navy and training exercises in, for example, the Royal Marines and the Parachute Brigade, in which the doctors are likely to be expected to share the active training, a prospect welcome to the vigorous and athletic.

Specialist services in all major disciplines, clinical, pathological and radiological, are maintained by the Armed Services, the small specialties on a collaborative basis between the Services, often supported by part-time civilian consultants. The peace keeping role of the Services and the relatively young age of service personnel ensures a greater demand for surgical specialties, and perhaps for psychiatry, than for medical specialties. With a good academic record, enthusiasm and drive there are relatively few but good opportunities for accredited specialist training in most major disciplines without the uncertainty and financial agony of finding suitable training posts in the NHS. Periods of secondment to eminent civilian units are usually arranged for special experience. At the end of specialist training most doctors, whether hospital doctors or general practitioners return to civilian life; only a small proportion rise to senior rank and a permanent career in the Armed Forces.

Medical cadetships, which provide on a competitive basis, a full maintenance grant and tuition fees during undergraduate clinical education in return for a five-year commitment to serve in the sponsoring branch of the Services after full registration, are a convenient and common path of entry. Other doctors take short-service commissions for three or five years on completion of preregistration post and leave with a useful tax-free gratuity to assist in the transition back to civilian life. A few but exciting opportunities exist for research into aspects such as aviation medicine and underwater medicine in Service establishments.

The Armed Forces offer recent graduates potentially wide opportunities and security at a very insecure moment in their careers. The difficulty, if planning to specialise in anything other than general practice, is to acquire precisely the desired specialist training. Whatever else, the absolute prerequisite is a liking for Service life.

Journalism

For centuries occasional medical graduates have become accomplished authors and playwrights. Medicine's window into hearts and lives is a good springboard to fiction. Fiction apart, medicine has high profile public interest and a substantial demand exists for good, readable informed medical writing, broadcasts and television. Few are born writers but many learn by experience; a formal journalistic training is not probably what a doctor who wants to write and can write needs. Most start by writing and selling an article or two and are then asked for more by nonmedical or medical newspapers. The art of compiling and managing a medical journal is different but of course not altogether unrelated. Both the *British Medical Journal (BMJ)* and the *Lancet*, the two great British general medical journals, have vacancies for doctors from time to time. The *BMJ* and *BMJ News Review* also have imaginative schemes for student electives to give an introduction to medical journalism to a few students who have already shown flair. The editing of specialist medical journals, of which there are many published in Britain, is usually in the hands of an unpaid specialist editorial board or part-time medical editor with all the technical editing in nonmedical hands. Publishing offers a number of opportunities for doctors but the directors of many medical publishing organisations are not in fact medically trained.

Doctors and the Law

A number of doctors of a legal disposition and especially those who already have a legal qualification work for the Medical Defence organisations and a few become coroners. Coroners have to be either legally or medically qualified, many are both. Their job is responsible, important and interesting. Others become barristers, sometimes specialising in medical negligence. A few become judges.

Some doctors become famous musicians and conductors, which speaks to the talented individuals who study medicine rather than indicating a hidden inspiration to music in medicine.

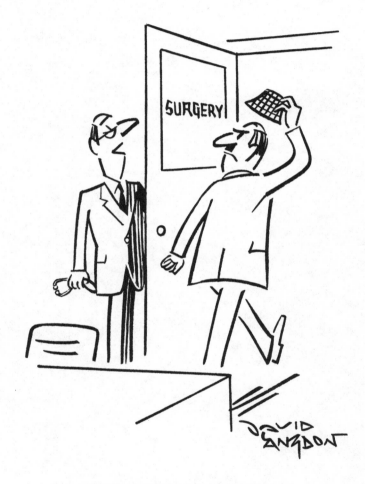

'By all means have a second opinion.
Call in tomorrow and I'll give you one ...'

12

The beginning of the end: independent practice

The stress of achievement

It is very good to arrive. Arriving is not, however, without its own stresses. The journey has been hard, long and uncertain. We are told that about half of medical graduates at one time or another during their training regret having gone into medicine[3] but there are no control figures for other occupations, so does that really mean much at all? The fact remains that the great majority are pleased and fulfilled when they arrive. The grass is greener once the post is permanent and the status independent. Salary may not immediately increase, especially in hospital because consultants do not get extra duty payments. In any walk of life, however, it is necessary to be prepared for the experience that to achieve one's ambition can be an unsettling even disturbing experience after long years of expectation, a feeling vividly captured in another context by David Holbrook on becoming a Fellow of King's College, Cambridge:

> For some (and for all of us some of the time) the satisfactions of attainment are intolerable, and the exigencies of creative maturity unacceptable. When a dream is fulfilled it at once becomes part of mortal, time-ridden, mutable and mundane life: it must be disillusioned to be true. Such change presents us with a need to deal with an imperfect, intractable and troublesome actuality about which we have hitherto dreamt.

Final and often somewhat uncertain clinical decisions are now yours. Making decisions can be a lonely business especially in general practice. A sense of humility even of inadequacy is quite natural, even healthy, but may be painful. Junior staff expect and need a decisive leader. Patients want sympathetic but firm explanations and confident action.

Work becomes more peripatetic: outpatient clinics are often held at more than one location, in country districts often at a distance, interrupting the continuity of care a consultant can give to seriously ill inpatients. Slowly but surely as commitments increase the consultant is edged out of the front line of inpatient care by the junior staff, for it simply is not possible to be everywhere at once, but the final responsibility is the consultant's.

Always be prepared to ask a colleague for a second opinion. Second opinions provide interest as well as help. Welcome, even suggest a second opinion on the rare occasions when patients or relatives clearly doubt the correctness of diagnosis or management. Sir Cyril Clothier made a plea for second opinions without umbrage:

> When one receives the bad news of disaster to oneself or to someone very close, there is an instinctive reaching out for reassurance and confirmation as to even the most redoubtable opinion. This is an entirely natural and spontaneous reaction, which should on no account be mistaken for a lack of respect for the opinion already received. It is indeed a weakness for any professional person to resent a request for a second opinion.[8]

The temptation at any level of seniority in medicine to temper uncertainty with arrogance must be firmly resisted.

Teamwork between hospitals and general practice

Consultants are no less busy than junior medical staff (at least during the day) but are busy in different ways. New consultants are tried out by the local general practitioners on outpatients and on domiciliary visits. Domiciliary visits are worth more than the rapid clinical diagnosis they provide and possibly an avoided admission to hospital. They are worth the time and trouble because they help general practitioners and consultants to develop a working partnership, to learn from each other's different attitudes, experiences and perspectives. The best clinical practice is teamwork, and that includes teamwork between doctors in hospital and outside. It is so often revealing to see the patient in his or her human setting, as general practitioners know well. Examining patients without the trappings of hospital is an educational experience for consultants. Anyone who, armed with ophthalmoscope, has chased an unwilling patient (who turned out to have a cerebral tumour) around a double bed in quest of his optic discs will know how much more difficult examination can be at home. Even taking a history is more difficult with all the distraction of worried relatives, noisy children and domestic animals.

Visiting patients at home gives the countryside or town a new and human face. Houses, cottages and farms take on their own identities, associations, memories of illness won and lost. It brings a feeling of belonging and mattering to the community, which general practitioners experience early but most hospital doctors have not had the opportunity to discover.

Administrative responsibilities

In laboratory-based disciplines, becoming a consultant brings more administrative responsibility: more time managing the service and staff, less at the bench; and sooner or later there is a departmental budget to balance. Consultants find themselves spending too much time at administrative meetings, mostly frustrating because they result in no executive action. The introduction of clinical resource management to all services in the hospital provides an opportunity for an effective medical input into management; the administrative load will be greater on some than before but the results should justify the effort.

Continuing education

Invitations will come to address postgraduate meetings, initially to try you out as well as to hear what you have to say. After a few years as a consultant you may be invited to become the hospital's clinical tutor or, as a general practitioner, the GP Tutor – both interesting and important roles in the gift of the Regional Post-graduate Dean and carrying overall responsibility for the post-graduate centre and its educational programme. All consultants have a responsibility to keep up-to-date and to teach their junior staff. Playing an active part in the postgraduate education pro-gramme of the hospital is an inherent part of their responsibility and not an optional extra to be submerged by other activities however worthy. Consultants are now nominated as the 'edu-cational supervisors' of individual members of the junior staff – a professional and, at best, a partly pastoral role requiring both time and effort.

Besides the daily demands of providing a service, educating and counselling junior colleagues (who need opportunities to discuss their progress and future), possibly continuing in clinical re-search, and being part of family and local community, the doctor has somehow to keep up-to-date with a rapidly changing subject. Not many years after obtaining a career post in any field the realisation dawns that the knowledge and skill, recently so bright and up-to-date is slowly but steadily tarnishing. Keeping it polished is a major challenge, a problem and sometimes a burden. The core of practice remains the same from year to year: patients change little and most ill health continues to have unsophisticated causes. But therapeutics is changing fast. Are innovations real advances or simply expensive well advertised variations on a theme? Are new diagnostic techniques an essential aid to effective daily practice or is their risk and cost only justified in very specific and rare circumstances? What is fashion, what is fad?

At least one general medical journal should be taken and read. Better to read one regularly, promptly and thoughtfully than to let several pile up expensive, erudite and unopened. Do not bite off more than you can chew but do chew what you bite. There is much to be said also for reading at least one specialist journal.

Clinical meetings are an important source of education for senior staff as well as for juniors; for general practitioners as well as for hospital doctors. It should be a matter of honour between colleagues to attend and to ensure that time and trouble is taken over one's own team's presentations. Meetings attended by all the staff always provide a worthwhile educational workshop with something for everyone, but as soon as individuals begin to fall

out for gold, golf or simply through bad organisation, part of the
breadth of institutional expertise is lost, disillusionment sets in
and the whole endeavour founders.

It is easier to keep up as one of a team and as part of an
institution. The hardest setting in which to keep up is in single-
handed practice. Continuing education, revision of existing
knowledge and continued cultivation of a critical interest in the
gaps in knowledge are essential background to good practice.
New discoveries and failing memory require determined and
consistent effort.

Private practice

One of the attractions of private clinical practice is that it main-
tains a personal one-to-one relationship with patients which it is
difficult to retain with the wide responsibility and teamwork of
NHS practice. The decision whether or not to undertake private
practice depends on personal inclination and location. In the large
cities and the South, private practice may be financially very
rewarding; in surgical specialties and in obstetrics and gynaecology it is not difficult to earn the basic NHS salary several times
over without encroaching on time contracted to the NHS.

Fulltime NHS consultants are permitted to earn up to 10% of
their gross salary in private practice without foregoing any NHS
pay. If they earn more, they forfeit one-eleventh of their NHS
salary, a relatively small sacrifice but enough to make it necessary
to calculate the advantage and disadvantage carefully in low-
earning specialties or in areas where the demand for private
practice is small, so as to ensure that after deduction of expenses
the time and effort is worthwhile.

The main problem with private practice is to control it. Its
insistent demands can easily erode a full personal service to NHS
patients, price out of the market the time formerly spent on
teaching, research and keeping up-to-date and seriously interrupt
evenings and weekends. Private practice intrudes far less if
centred on the private wing of an NHS hospital but few NHS
hospitals have suitable inpatient and outpatient accommodation.
Private practice offers nothing over the NHS in quality of service,

only in convenience, comfort and personal attention from the consultant. What it normally fails to provide is the continuous cover by junior staff on site who in the NHS ensure that emergencies are instantly dealt with day and night. To be involved in private practice completes the social mix of a consultant's practice: many doctors enjoy serving poor and rich alike and find it as unacceptable to deny their services to someone who wants to pay as to someone who cannot.

The private practice dilemma also confronts university staff but to a lesser degree. Traditionally, clinical academics have not been permitted by their universities to charge patients and keep the money. Personal gain from private clinical practice has been seen as too great a threat to the essential teaching and research function. Recently, under economic pressure and out of a wish to see broad equivalence between the pay of clinical academics and fulltime NHS staff, a 10% rule similar to that applied to fulltime NHS consultant staff has been introduced by several universities, on the condition that private practice is confined to the university hospital and that the time spent is strictly limited.

Academic units have long provided service on a team basis to all sections of the population, including patients from abroad not entitled to treatment under the NHS. The service to private patients has been part of a complete service or has arisen from the specialised interests of the unit and the research funds have benefited from the earnings. If the incentive of personal remuneration now drives the machine faster, teaching, research and the funding of research may suffer. More likely a new and reasonable equilibrium will be achieved. Private practice is a natural complement to the NHS and without detriment to it, provided that it does not divert scarce manpower resources (medical, nursing and other support services) from the NHS. Expanded to the point where the NHS was drained of expertise, private medicine would strike at the heart of the greatest social advance this country has ever seen. There is also a limit to which a doctor can effectively serve two masters, indeed three if a teaching role is included, as a consultant surgeon recently pointed out in a letter to the *BMJ*:

The commitment of the surgeon to any patient is comprehensive, but in private work the lack of junior colleagues means it can be heavy and unpredictable. It is unreasonable to call for more elective surgery to be performed in private hospitals and also to expect overextended surgeons to give as much time as they would wish to teaching and to out of hours emergency work in their NHS units.[26]

Private practice is a smaller issue in general practice. There are a few entirely private general practitioners but the great majority have only a handful of fee-paying patients, whose demands do not interfere with the care of NHS patients.

Privilege and responsibility

Through the rough and the smooth, it is a great privilege to have a job which matters to others, which does a great deal for a few and something for many. Those who do the small things conscientiously and consistently well can be trusted with the more complicated interventions. There is no more challenging and satisfying way of life, demanding and uncomfortable though medicine will always be. The compensation is to be working for a better future for individuals and better health of populations as a whole. Material rewards are reasonable, at least in permanent posts in the NHS, and high when combined with successful private practice: some doctors could have earned more in other walks of life – a number might have earned less.

Of course there are pitfalls:

> It was a very helpful feat
> To list the patients we must treat.
> In future issues let us see
> Presented categorically
> The kinds of docs we shouldn't be.
>
> First, the ambitious climber take,
> Who will department chairman make;
> Who toils to win professors' praise
> And quotes the journals phrase by phrase,
> But never reads the patients' gaze.

Next: the expert proud we find,
The latest savior to mankind.
Cured patients speak to his renown,
But he leaves sick ones with a frown,
Because they let his image down.

Third, the jovial friend of all,
Who never heard perfection's call.
His ken of medicine paper thin,
But patients' trust he'll always win:
They love him while he does them in.

And fourth, the well adjusted fellow,
Who seeks that all in life be mellow;
Who loves good music, wine and skis,
Resents his work but likes the fees,
And does not hear his patients' pleas.

To start the series, here are four,
But surely there are many more.
Just let us seek to see what's true
In what we are and what we do,
Lest we forget, we're human too.[27]

All said and done, it is marvellous to have arrived; to have the opportunity to set up a settled home and to begin to feel independent. But it is worth remembering that your memorial will be your kindness and thoroughness, which patients can assess, rather than your brilliance which, on the whole, they cannot; your ability to reassure about what they have not got as much as your ability to diagnose and treat potentially mortal disease. A letter from a friend whom I had referred to a most eminent doctor and clinical scientist said it all:

He says there is absolutely nothing wrong with me physically and as he spent over an hour and went into every avenue I believe him implicity.

I cannot tell you how much I appreciate your help, although the cause for the illness is not physical, it makes me feel very much better to know that it is not. I was beginning to think I was suffering from a mystery terminal illness.

To listen always, to help often and to cure sometimes, first during a long and demanding training and, finally, in a harmonious balance between professional and private life is the art of living medicine. There is no more challenging, worthwhile and fulfilling experience.

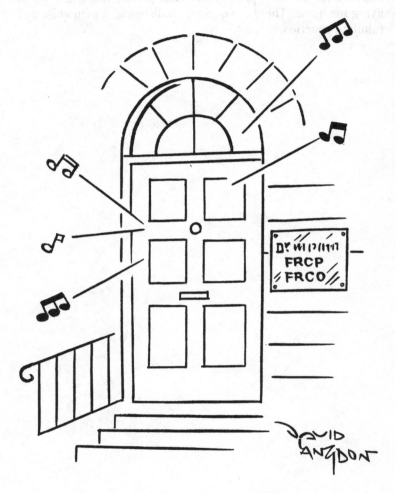

Some doctors become famous musicians ...

Appendix 1

General Medical Council Education Committee: Attributes of the Independent Practitioner

15. Joint Higher Training Committees, Royal Colleges and their Faculties have identified the aims of training in their own specialties. These include the acquisition of specialised knowledge and skill in the relevant preventive, clinical, laboratory, management, administrative, teaching or other fields to the point where the doctor is competent to accept and exercise the highest level of responsibility in a particular specialty.

16. Nevertheless, all doctors share a common role in the prevention or alleviation of disease or distress through appropriate intervention. Education and training for specialties should not only include acquisition of the technical knowledge and skills of a particular specialty or its branches, but also development of the attributes set out below; together they contribute to a doctor's professional development.

1 *The ability to solve clinical and other problems in medical practice*, which involves or requires:
(a) an intellectual and temperamental ability to change, to face the unfamiliar and to adapt to change;
(b) a capacity for individual, self-directed learning; and
(c) reasoning and judgement in the application of knowledge to the analysis and interpretation of data, in defining the nature of a problem, and in planning and implementing a strategy to resolve it.

2 *Possession of adequate knowledge and understanding of the general structure and function of the human body and workings of the mind, in health and disease, of their interaction and of the interaction between man and his physical and social environment.* This requires:
(a) knowledge of the physical, behavioural, epidemiological and clinical sciences upon which medicine depends;
(b) understanding of the aetiology and natural history of diseases;
(c) understanding of the impact of both psychological factors upon illness and of illness upon the patient and the patient's family;
(d) understanding of the effects of childhood growth and of later ageing upon the individual, the family and the community; and
(e) understanding of the social, cultural and environmental factors which contribute to health or illness, and the capacity of medicine to influence them.

3 *Possession of consultation skills*, which include:
(a) skills in sensitive and effective communication with patients and their families, professional colleagues and local agencies, and the keeping of good medical records;

(b) the clinical skills necessary to examine the patient's physical and mental state and to investigate appropriately;
(c) the ability to exercise sound clinical judgement to analyse symptoms and physical signs in pathophysiological terms, to establish diagnoses, and to offer advice to the patient taking account of physical, psychological, social and cultural factors; and
(d) understanding of the special needs of terminal care.

4 *Acquisition of a high standard of knowledge and skills in the doctor's specialty*, which include:
(a) understanding of acute illness and of disabling and chronic diseases within that specialty, including their physical, mental and social implications, rehabilitation, pain relief, and the need for support and encouragement; and
(b) relevant manual, biochemical, pharmacological, psychological, social and other interventions in acute and chronic illness.

5 *Willingness and ability to deal with common medical emergencies and with other illness in an emergency.*

6 *The ability to contribute appropriately to the prevention of illness and the promotion of health*, which involves:
(a) understanding of the principles, methods and limitations of preventive medicine and health promotion;
(b) understanding of the doctor's role in educating patients, families and communities, and in generally promoting good health; and
(c) the ability to identify individuals at risk and to take appropriate action.

7 *The ability to recognise and analyse ethical problems so as to enable patients, their families, society and the doctor to have proper regard to such problems in reaching decisions*; this comprehends:
(a) knowledge of the ethical standards and legal responsibilities of the medical profession;
(b) understanding of the impact of medico-social legislation on medical practice; and
(c) recognition of the influence upon his or her approach to ethical problems of the doctor's own personality and values.

8 *The maintenance of attitudes and conduct appropriate to a high level of professional practice*, which includes:
(a) recognition that a blend of scientific and humanitarian approaches is required, involving a critical approach to learning, open-mindedness, compassion, and concern for the dignity of the patient and, where relevant, of the patient's family;
(b) recognition that good medical practice depends on partnership between doctor and patient, based upon mutual understanding and trust; the doctor may give advice, but the patient must decide whether or not to accept it;

(c) commitment to providing high quality care; awareness of the limitations of the doctor's own knowledge and of existing medical knowledge; recognition of the duty to keep up to date in the doctor's own specialist field and to be aware of developments in others; and
(d) willingness to accept review, including self-audit, of the doctor's performance.

9 *Mastery of the skills required to work within a team and, where appropriate, assume the responsibilities of team leader,* which requires:
(a) recognition of the need for the doctor to collaborate in prevention, diagnosis, treatment and management with other health care professionals and with patients themselves;
(b) understanding and appreciation of the roles, responsibilities and skills of nurses and other health care workers; and
(c) the ability to lead, guide and co-ordinate the work of others.

10 *Acquisition of experience in administration and planning,* including:
(a) efficient management of the doctor's own time and professional activities;
(b) appropriate use of diagnostic and therapeutic resources, and appreciation of the economic and practical constraints affecting the provision of health care; and
(c) willingness to participate, as required, in the work of bodies which advise, plan and assist the development and administration of medical services, such as NHS authorities, Royal Colleges and Faculties, and professional associations.

11 *Recognition of the opportunities and acceptance of the duty to contribute, when possible, to the advancement of medical knowledge and skill,* which entails:
(a) understanding of the contribution of research methods, and interpretation and application of others' research in the doctor's own specialty; and
(b) willingness, when appropriate, to contribute to research in the doctor's specialist field, both personally and through encouraging participation by junior colleagues.

12 *Recognition of the obligation to teach others, particularly doctors in training,* which requires:
(a) acceptance of responsibility for training junior colleagues in the specialty, and for teaching other doctors, medical students, and other health care professionals, when required;
(b) recognition that teaching skills are not necessarily innate but can be learned, and willingness to acquire them; and
(c) recognition that the example of the teacher is the most powerful influence upon the standards of conduct and practice of every trainee.

From: General Medical Council Education Committee
      Recommendations on the Training of Specialists.
      London, 1987

Appendix 2
Estimated minimum duration of specialist training and the timing of higher diplomas and/or specialist accredition (see text Chapter 4 for proposed changes).

Training Phases	Basic Medical Education		Specialist Training							
		General Clinical Training	General Professional Training/Basic Specialist Training			Higher Specialist Training				
Years	1 – 5 or 1 – 6	6	7	8	9	10	11	12	13	14
Psychiatry	→	PRELIM			MRCPsych				No accreditation	
Anaesthetics (i)	→	PRIMARY			FFARCS			ACCRED		
Obstetrics/ Gynaecology (ii)	→				MRCOG			ACCRED		
Pathology (iii)	→		Pt I	MRCPath			MRCPath	No accreditation		
Radiology/ Radiotherapy	→		Pt I	FRCR			FRCR	ACCRED		
General Surgery/Surgical Specialties (except as under noted) (Eng)	→	PRIMARY			FRCS			ACCRED		
Surgery/Surgical Specialties (except as under noted) (Edin)	→	PRIMARY			FRCS			ACCRED		
General Surgery & Surgical Specialties (Glasg)	→	PRIMARY			FRCS			ACCRED		
Oral/Maxillofacial Surgery (Edin) (iv)	→	PRIMARY	FRCS					ACCRED		
Otolaryngology/ Plastic Surgery	→	PRIMARY			FRCS			ACCRED		
General Practice	→				MRCGP					
General Practice (Vocational training for)	→				CPE					
General (Internal) Medicine	→	MRCP			MRCP			ACCRED		
Medical Specialties (Except as shown below)	→	MRCP			MRCP			ACCRED		
Accident & Emergency Medicine	→	MRCP		FRCS	MFRCS FARCS			ACCRED		(v)
Community Medicine	→	MRCP	Pt I	MFC	Pt II	MFC			ACCRED	(vi)
Occupational Medicine	→	MRCP			AFOM			ACCRED MFOM		(vii)
Haematology	→	MRCP		Pt I	MRCPath	MRCP		MRCPath	ACCRED	
Communicable Diseases	→	MRCP			MRCP			ACCRED		
Genitourinary Medicine	→	MRCP			MRCOG MRCP			ACCRED		

NOTES:

(i) Must be age 25 or over for conferral of FFARCS.

(ii) Can enter specialist training with Part I MRCOG provided that the Part II training requirements have been completed.

(iii) Part II MRCPath written papers can be taken after 3 years' training, but the practical/orals only after 5 years' training.

(iv) Candidates are required to possess registrable medical and dental qualifications. FRCS at year 8 only if candidate has 1 year's experience in approved posts in oral and maxillo-facial surgery, after obtaining a dental degree but prior to a medical degree.

(v) The thesis for Membership may be submitted at any time within 3 years of passing Part I. Higher specialist training commences when a senior registrar post has been secured. Membership, & 4 years' higher specialist training are required for accreditation.

(vi) MFOM required for accreditation.

(vii) MRCPath required for accreditation.

(viii) In medicine/medical specialties the information given relates to accreditation in single/dual specialties. For triple accreditation, 6 years' higher medical training is required.

(ix) The earliest point at which MRCP can be obtained has been shown.

Adapted from General Medical Education Recommendations on the Training of Specialists London (1987).

Appendix 3
Study leave

Definition

250. Professional or study leave is granted for postgraduate purposes approved by the employing authority, and includes study (usually, but not exclusively or necessarily, on a course), research, teaching, examining or taking examinations, visiting clinics and attending professional conferences.

Recommended standard for professional and study leave in the United Kingdom

251. Subject to the conditions in paragraph 254, professional or study leave will normally be granted to the maximum extent consistent with maintaining essential services in accordance with the recommended standards, or may exceptionally be granted under the provisions of paragraph 252. The recommended standards are:

a. Consultants
   SHMOs and SHDOs
   ASs
   Hospital practitioners
Leave with pay and expenses, with a maximum of thirty days (including off-duty days falling within the period of leave) in any period of three years for professional purposes within the United Kingdom.
b. SRs
In addition to an aggregate, normally equivalent to at least one day per week for individual study and specific research projects, professional leave with pay and expenses within a maximum of an annual rate of ten days over a period of three years; this allowance being cumulative over three years, provided that the total amount due in three years is not taken until one year of the appointment has been served. This allowance may be carried over within the three year period on promotion to a permanent post in grades listed at a. above.
c. Rs
   SHOs
   HOs and post-registration medical HOs
   i. Practitioners in these grades should receive either day release with pay and expenses for the equivalent of one day a week during Uni-

versity terms; or leave with pay and expenses within a maximum calculated at a rate of thirty days in a year (the year for this purpose being counted from 1 October). This allowance may accumulate over the period of the appointment, provided that the total amount due in the period of appointment is not taken until one year of the appointment has been served.

ii. Such practitioners may also receive leave with pay and expenses (other than examination fees) for the purpose of sitting an examination for a higher qualification, except that, where the authority considers that this would be contrary to the interests of the individual or the service, leave may be refused (for example, repeated sitting and failing of the same examination could be held to be an unjustifiable use of paid leave). Expenses may be paid only where taking the examination is the natural culmination of a course of study approved by the authority.

d. Pre-registration HOs should be allowed reasonable time within working hours for attending, within the hospital, clinico-pathological conferences and ward rounds with other firms.

Additional periods of professional and study leave in the United Kingdom

252. Authorities may at their discretion grant professional or study leave in the United Kingdom above the periods recommended in paragraph 251 with or without pay and with or without expenses or with some proportion thereof.

Professional and study leave outside the United Kingdom

253. Authorities may at their discretion grant professional or study leave outside the United Kingdom with or without pay and with or without expenses or with any proportion thereof.

Conditions

254. The following conditions shall apply:

a. where a practitioner is employed by more than one authority, the leave and the purpose for which it is required must be approved by all the authorities concerned;

b. where leave with pay is granted, the practitioner must not undertake any remunerative work without the special permission of the leave-granted authority;

c. where an application is made under paragraphs 252 or 253 for a period of leave with pay, and this exceeds three weeks, it shall be open to the authority to require that one half of the excess over three weeks shall be counted against annual leave entitlement, the carry forward or anticipation of annual leave within a maximum of three weeks being permitted for this purpose (this condition shall not be applied to practitioners attending certain courses of specialist training notified to authorities for this purpose by the Department).

From: *Hospital Medical and Dental Staff (England and Wales);*
Terms and Conditions of Service. National Health Service (1986).

Appendix 4
Useful addresses for further information on specialty examination regulations and requirements

Royal Colleges and Faculties

College of Anaesthetists, 35–43 Lincoln's Inn Fields, London WC2A 3PN

Faculty of Community Medicine of the Royal College of Physicians of the United Kingdom, 28 Portland Place, London W1N 4DE

Faculty of Occupational Medicine, Royal College of Physicians, 11 St Andrews Place, London NW1 4LE

Royal College of General Practitioners, 14 Prince's Gate, London SW7 1PU

Royal College of Obstetricians and Gynaecologists, 27 Sussex Place, London NW1 4RG

Royal College of Pathologists, 2 Carlton House Terrace, London SW1Y 5AF

Royal College of Physicians, 11 St Andrew's Place, London NW1 4LE

Royal College of Physicians of Edinburgh, 9 Queen Street, Edinburgh EH2 1JQ

Royal College of Physicians and Surgeons of Glasgow, 234–42 St Vincent Street, Glasgow G2 5RJ

Royal College of Psychiatrists, 17 Belgrave Square, London SW1X 8PG

Royal College of Radiologists, 38 Portland Place, London W1N 3DG

Royal College of Surgeons of Edinburgh, 18 Nicholson Street, Edinburgh EH8 9DW

Royal College of Surgeons of England, 35–43 Lincoln's Inn Fields, London WC2A 3PN

Armed Forces medical services

RAMC Officer Recruiting Team, Regimental Headquarters RAMC, Royal Army Medical College, Millbank, London SW1P 4RJ

The Medical Director General (Naval), (Attention Med P1(N)), Ministry of Defence, First Avenue House, 40–8 High Holborn, London WC1Y 6HE

Ministry of Defence MA1 (RAF), First Avenue House, High Holborn, London WC1V 6HE

Medical defence organisations

The Medical Defence Union, 3 Devonshire Place, London W1N 2EA
The Medical and Dental Society of Scotland, James Sellars House, 144
   West George Street, Glasgow G22 8W
The Medical Protection Society, 50 Hallam Street, London W1N 6DE

Other organisations

British Medical Association, BMA House, Tavistock Square, London
   WC1 9JP
General Medical Council, 44 Hallam Street, London W1N 6AE
Medical Practitioners Union, 10 Jamestown Road, London NW1
Medical Research Council, 20 Park Crescent, London W1N 4AL
Medical Women's Federation, BMA House, Tavistock Square, London
   WC1 9JP

References

1 Richards, P. (1989). *Learning medicine 1990*, 6th edn. London: British Medical Association.
2 DHSS Medical Manpower and Education Division (1988). Medical and dental staffing prospects in the NHS in England and Wales in 1987. *Health Trends*, 20, 101–9.
3 Allen, I. (1988). *Doctors and their careers*. London: Policy Studies Institute.
4 Parkhouse, J., Campbell, M. G. & Parkhouse, H. F. (1983). Career preferences of doctors qualifying in 1974–80: a comparison of pre-registration findings. *Health Trends*, 15, 29–35.
5 University Hospitals Association of England and Wales (1989). *The Early Postgraduate Years*. Leeds.
6 DHSS (1987). *Hospital medical staffing: achieving a balance – plan for action*. London.
7 Paget, J. (1869). What becomes of medical students. *St. Bartholomew's Hospital Reports*, 5, 238–42.
8 Clothier, C. (1987). *The patient's dilemma*. London: Nuffield Provincial Hospitals Trust.
9 Hampton, J. R. (1983). The end of clinical freedom. *British Medical Journal*, 287, 1237–8.
10 McCaughey, D. (1988). Arthur E. Mills Memorial Oration given at the Golden Jubilee Meeting of the Royal Australasian College of Physicians, Sydney, 9th May, 1988.
11 American College of Physicians Ethics Mannual (1984). Part 11: Research, other ethical issues. *Annals of Internal Medicine*, 101, 263–74.
12 Hoffenberg, R. (1986). *Clinical Freedom*. London: Nuffield Provincial Hospitals Trust.
13 Brahams, D. (1985). Doctor's duty to inform patients of substantial or special risks when offering treatment. *Lancet*, 1, 528–30.
14 General Medical Council (1987). *Professional conduct and discipline: fitness to practise*. London.
15 Anonymous (1841). The Physiology of the London Medical Student: 7. Of various other diverting matters concerned with grinding. *Punch*, 1, 213.
16 Anonymous (1841). The Physiology of the London Medical Student: 9. Of the sequel to the Examination Hall. *Punch*, 1, 229.

17   General Medical Council (1987). *Recommendations on General Clinical Training*. London.
18   Bogdonoff, M. D. (1987). Educational consequences of changing medical responsibility in university hospitals. *New England Journal of Medicine*, 317, 765–6.
19   Stanley, G. *Sunday Times*. September 11, 1988.
20   Parkhouse, J. & Ellin, D. J. (1988). Reasons for doctors' career choice and change of choice. *British Medical Journal*, 296, 1651–3.
21   Black, D. A. K. (1984) *An Anthology of False Antitheses*. London: Nuffield Provincial Hospitals Trust.
22   Medawar, P. B. (1979). *Advice to a Young Scientist*. New York: Harper and Row.
23   Women in Medicine. (1987). *Careers for Women in Medicine: Planning and Pitfalls*. Newcastle-on-Tyne: Women in Medicine. (Obtainable from Women in Medicine, 7c Cassland Road, London E9)
24   Bishop, W. J. (1953). The evolution of the general practitioner in England. In *Science, Medicine and History*, I, ed. E. A. Underwood, pp. 351–7. London: Oxford University Press.
25   Report of the Committee of Inquiry into the Future Development of the Public Health Function (1988). *Public Health in England*. London: HMSO.
26   Jones, P. F. (1988). Letter. *British Medical Journal*, 296, 1600.
27   Brotschi, E. (1978). Letter. *New England Journal of Medicine*, 299, 367.

Further reading

How to do it 1. London:BMJ., £6.95 (BMA members £6.45)
How to do it 2. London:BMJ., £6.95 (BMA members £6.45)
Procedures in Practice, 2nd edn. London:BMJ., £6.95 (BMA members £6.45)
A Sense of Asher. London: BMJ., £7.00 (BMA members £6.50)

Index

Printed in the United States
by Bookmasters

Printed in the United States
By Bookmasters